DATE DUE

DEMCO, INC. 38-2931

CANCER: We Live and Die by Radiation

CANCER
We Live and Die by Radiation

Michelangelo Delfino

and

Mary E. Day

MoBeta Publishing
United States

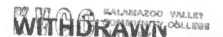

MoBeta Publishing
Los Altos, CA 94023-0571
www.mobeta.com

SAN 254-9050

Copyright © 2006 by MoBeta, Inc.

Library of Congress Control Number 2006927973

ISBN 0972514112

Printed in the United States of America
First Printing August 2006

Preface

This is a book about radiation oncology, a study of cancer and the role radiation plays in its development, diagnosis, and treatment. This book explores radiation as both a killer and a healer by introducing the reader to the effect of radiation on the body and the way radiation is harnessed to both diagnose and destroy cancer.

After introducing the tools used for diagnosis and treatment, a brief explanation is given on how cancer is measured using staging and statistics. Who gets cancer and the risk factors for each particular cancer are briefly described with comparisons made between the United States, Canada, Japan, and the U.K. Cancers are then individually described and grouped somewhat arbitrarily by body site and function.

The discussions of each cancer include summaries of key trials and recent studies of modern treatment options by stage focusing on the efficacy of radiotherapy and its associated risks with comparisons to alternative therapies such as surgery and chemotherapy. Each chapter concludes with practical evaluations of the "best treatment" with an emphasis on quality of life. The use of radiation for palliation and treating other diseases is also described.

This work is written with the patient, the family, the friends, and the caregivers in mind for the purpose of providing a quick reference for making informed choices. Knowledge of science is not necessary as concepts are defined in simple terms and easy access is provided for important information such as cancer staging, cancer statistics, radiography and radiotherapy tools, radiotherapy techniques, and radionuclides used in brachytherapy. For those interested in further research, references to original works are included. The book includes a glossary and an appendix.

The authors are former research scientists who collectively spent nearly three decades working at Varian Medical Systems, a publicly traded corporation where they invented implantable radioactive medical devices and novel X-ray tube technologies. After Varian they founded a research and development start-up company that marketed a new brachytherapy source to treat restenosis and other diseases. Since then the authors have been struggling with their own recurring basal cell carcinomas as two of America's medically uninsured.

The authors are grateful to the physicians, nurses, scientists, and staff who generously provided copies of published work and other writings. Here, any failure, omission, or error is solely the responsibility of the authors. *Cancer: We Live and Die by Radiation* is their second book.

Michelangelo Delfino, Ph.D. and Mary E. Day
16 August 2006

Contents

Once Upon a Time

Cancer is a disease—an abnormal condition that accounts for some 13% of all deaths in the world. Second to heart disease as a cause of death, cancer is arguably this planet's most frightening killer. No one is spared— cancer threatens every man, woman, and child, even the unborn. The disease has no fear and knows no global boundaries.

> The risk of getting cancer is higher in the developed world, but cancers in the developing world are more fatal. Overall, the probability for an individual of dying from cancer during their lifetime is not very different in the developed and developing world. (Mackay et al. 2006, 44-45)

At the turn of the new millennium, the World Health Organization estimated that 6.2 million men, women, and children had died of cancer in the year 2000. This 192 member United Nations organization went on to predict that the number of people who would die from cancer would grow to 7.6 million in 2005, to 9 million in 2015, and to 11.4 million in 2030, and with no end in sight (Stewart and Kleihues 2003).   There are some people in the medical community, like the head of the National Cancer Institute (NCI) in the United States who believe otherwise:

> You recently announced a goal ... the elimination of "death and suffering" from cancer by the year 2015. Why 12 years from now? It's not a magic moment, obviously. Hopefully, we will do it sooner. But 2015 was what I believed was a realistic target, given the progress we are making in the laboratory. (National Cancer Institute 2003)

Perhaps the NCI is right, but for now, no part of the human body that replicates is immune from cancer—hair, teeth, and nails do not reproduce and they do not get cancer.   In people, there are more than 200 different cancers, each one assigned to a specific organ like the lung and breast, or a type of tissue like the skin and bone, and 40% of these cancers are thought to be preventable.

Surviving cancer is sometimes no less terrifying than actually succumbing to it as very often a part of the person's body must be removed for survival and this loss may go far deeper than any scar. Even when the battle for life is won and the disease is seemingly removed, cancer has a nasty habit of recurring and returning with a vengeance that often destroys more than just its human target with a toll that truly taxes everyone including the caregivers as one such physician so eloquently expressed:

> an unremitting sense of sadness, helplessness and guilt that while trying to do something to heal, the doctor turned out to be the mundane instrument that helped usher an exemplary human being from the world. (Peschel and Peschel 1990)

Risk factors are conditions that promote cancer and fuel its rage. These variables are known to increase the probability of developing cancer but are not necessarily responsible for causing it. There are two kinds of cancer risk factors. Age, genetics, race, sex, and height are universal ones to which we are predisposed and cannot change. In a sense they reflect the randomness, excitement, and unfairness of life itself. Other risk factors are preventable in that they are subject to human intervention. These risk factors include things like obesity, low fruit and vegetable intake, physical inactivity, consumption of addictive substances—smoking and alcohol, practice of unsafe sex, exposure to urban air pollution, indoor smoke from household use of solid fuels, and use of contaminated injections in health care settings which are said to contribute to over one third of all worldwide cancer deaths (Danaei et al. 2005).

Radiation is a special risk factor because it is both universal—naturally occurring, and specific—artificially produced. The National Academy of Sciences (2006) estimates that approximately 18% of America's exposure to radiation is from artificially produced sources. This duality, however, was not always so, in that artificially created radiation is relatively new, in fact it is a late 19th century European invention that ironically preceded the first observation of natural radiation by one year. With its discovery came a new wave of cancer victims and cancer treatment methodologies that demanded caution:

> Cancer patients are lied to, not just because the disease is (or is thought to be) a death sentence, but because it is felt to be obscene — in the original meaning of that word: ill-omened, abominable, repugnant to the senses. (Sontag 2001, 9)

You see, even though exposure to radiation was always considered dangerous, it is possible that no one explained to the controversial American essayist that the massive doses of radiation used to treat one cancer would some 30 years later be the likely the cause of her death from another. And while cancer and radiation are as deadly as ever, their unusual relationship makes for a unique interplay that is the subject of this book.

A Tale of Two Killers

We cannot see it and we certainly do not feel it. And yet radiation is everywhere—it cannot be avoided—even the air we breathe is radioactive as is the ground we walk on. Moreover, the human body itself is radioactive as is every other living thing. If this were not enough, our planet is constantly bombarded by cosmic rays from outer space. Admittedly, while exposure to natural sources of radiation is at an extremely low level, it does contribute to a lifelong dose of radiation that has cumulative consequences.

So should we be concerned with voluntarily exposing ourselves to a little bit more of this invisible stuff?

Science 101

Radiation collectively refers to particles that travel at the speed of light—186,000 miles per second—and have no mass. Mass is a fundamental property of all materials and is proportional to weight. Also called photons, radiation encompasses an energy spectrum (range of energies—energy is the capacity to do work, to produce or absorb heat) that includes cosmic rays, gamma rays, X-rays, ultraviolet (UV) light, visible light, infrared (IR) light, microwaves, and radio waves. Cosmic rays, for example, are the most energetic (fastest vibrating) and radio waves the least.

In space where there is nothing, a photon travels forever and that is why the concept of a light year (distance light travels in a year) is a useful measurement. In materials, photons are absorbed sooner or later. Low energy photons are more easily absorbed than high energy ones and materials composed of so-called light elements (atoms with few electrons, e.g., carbon) are more easily penetrated than those composed of heavier elements (e.g., lead) and of course a greater number of atoms means more mass and a higher rate of absorption. A nominal ½-inch thick lead plate, for example, is equivalent to 3 inches of concrete or about 600 feet of air in stopping gamma rays.

A photon that is not absorbed by a material is either transmitted through it or reflected away from it. There is no other possibility. If the photon has sufficient energy it can ionize the atoms—literally dislodge the electrons out of the atoms it contacts—in the material irradiated and thus create charged particles. Higher energy of photons can cause more ionization than lower energy photons.

The Little Cell that Could

The human body is organic (carbon-based) and estimated to have 100,000,000,000,000 cells. Each cell, while teaming with a myriad of chemicals, is mostly water and water is a remarkable molecule (combination of two hydrogen atoms and one oxygen atom) that is easily ionized.

Ionization temporarily causes water and any other ionizable molecules inside the cell to become more reactive than normal whereupon they can effect a change in the cell's genetic material—deoxyribonucleic acid (DNA). This extremely complex molecule (a seemingly endless combination of hydrogen, carbon, nitrogen, oxygen, and phosphorus atoms), if damaged and not repaired, may reproduce to become a cancerous cell.

Exposing a living cell to ionizing radiation always causes it some harm even if it is just a one-time event. On January 31, 2005, the United States issued this warning:

> X-ray radiation and gamma-radiation are listed in the report as 'known human carcinogens' because human studies show that exposure to these kinds of radiation causes many types of cancer including leukemia and cancers of the thyroid, breast and lung. (National Institute of Environmental Health Sciences 2005a)

The National Cancer Institute has long pointed out that at any point in time a damaged cell is capable of mutating (permanently changing the DNA) and once mutated the probability increases that cancer will develop sometime thereafter (Boice Jr. 1981). This rather alarming cellular alteration can occur with cosmic rays, gamma rays, X-rays, and the shortest wavelength UV radiation, all of which are ionizing forms of radiation:

> Of the estimated worldwide exposure to X-radiation and gamma radiation, about 43% is from natural sources, about 55% is from medical diagnosis and treatment with all other sources contributing to less than 2%. (National Institute of Environmental Health Sciences 2005b)

What makes cancer a so frightening and so formidable disease is that cancer is caused by the mutation of a single cell–but one in which the mutated cell behaves almost as if it were immortal, never ceasing to reproduce and never reaching maturity until the disease literally takes over the whole body.

A Special Relationship

Radiation sickness, literally a poisoning of the body, is another consequence of exposure to excess ionizing radiation. The exposure may be acute or chronic. Acute exposure is a one-time exposure to a very high level of radiation. Chronic exposure is cumulative, a long-term exposure to a low level of radiation. And while radiation sickness may not necessarily lead to cancer, there is no treatment that can reverse the cellular damage caused by the radiation. The irradiated person either recovers or dies.

The symptoms of radiation sickness can include weakness, nausea, dehydration, diarrhea, hair loss, inflammation, ulceration, and bleeding. The medical practitioners who deal with cancer patients undergoing radiation therapy (also called radiotherapy) often simply refer to these symptoms as "side effects" because they ultimately disappear after exposure ends. The harm, however, may remain, for the severity of this illness depends largely on the amount of radiation that has been deposited in the body. The absorbed dose is measured in units of Gray (Gy)–the energy deposited per unit mass. One Gy is also equivalent to 100 rem or 1 Sievert (Sv).

A one-time exposure to 450 Gy of ionizing radiation is sufficient to kill the average adult within days or weeks and the National Academy of Sciences (2006) warns that every Gy will increase the incidence of cancer by 8%. However, even a lower radiation dose can be detrimental:

> Estimates of risk should be limited to individuals receiving a dose of 5 rem [0.05 Gy] in one year or a lifetime dose of 10 rem [0.1 Gy] in addition to natural background [radiation]. (Health Physics Society 2004)

As a point of reference, the inescapable natural background radiation from outer space, rock, soil, air, people, plants, animals, and other naturally radioactive sources averages 0.004 Gy (or 0.4 rem) per year. Background radiation varies from place to place. For example, the mile high city, Denver, has about twice the cosmic ray dose of Los Angeles, which is at sea level.

And while no one seems to know, or at least agree on, the minimum dose required to cause cancer in humans, the medical community is advised to "reduce radiation dose ... as low as reasonably achievable (ALARA)" (Semelka 2006) or in other words, to be as prudent as possible.

Every cell is at risk, and some cells —such as those in the gonads (ovaries and testes)—are more sensitive to ionizing radiation than those in the skin or breast. Young cells are particularly sensitive to ionization because they are more actively dividing. This makes them more likely to mutate and possibly become cancerous:

> The risk of developing cancers due to these forms of ionizing radiation depends to some extent on age at the time of exposure. Childhood exposure is linked to an increased risk for leukemia and thyroid cancer. (National Institute of Environmental Health Sciences 2005a)

Although, cancer is uncommon in childhood, it is according to the National Cancer Institute, the second most likely cause of death in children up to 14 years old (Zahm and Devesa 1995). Leukemia and brain cancer are the two most common cancers in children, accounting for half of all newly diagnosed cases. Childhood cancers have been linked to intrauterine (in the womb) radiation exposure in both the United States and the U.K. (Doll and Wakeford 1997; Boice Jr. and Miller 1999). A study of upstate New Yorkers demonstrated that pediatric thyroid cancer is associated with exposure to ionizing radiation in infancy, especially in Jewish female children (Hempelmann et al. 1975). A Swedish study found that the risk of thyroid cancer developing as much as 15 years after exposure to X-rays is greater in children than in adults (Damber 2002).

And while no cancer is uniquely induced by ionizing radiation, it is almost universally accepted that cancer can result from a single exposure to ionizing radiation with risk increasing with dose:

> Ionizing radiation has been shown to induce (cause) cancer in many different species of animals and in almost all parts of the body. It is one of the few scientifically proven carcinogens (cancer-causing) agents in human beings…. The probability that cancer will result from radiation exposure increases as the dose increases. (American Cancer Society 2006b)

Since 1946, the American Cancer Society (2005a) has "invested about $3 billion in cancer research." And yet, in spite of its findings, in spite of its warnings concerning the risks of exposure to radiation, and in spite of the actions of a relatively prudent medical community, some scientists argue that a low-dose of ionizing radiation may in fact be harmless. Some scientists even suggest that although ionizing radiation damages the DNA, the DNA is soon repaired by stimulating the body's defense mechanisms (Cuttler 2004; Cuttler and Pollycove 2003). The argument these scientists propose is similar to the medical basis for vaccination—prepare the body for a life-and-death war by engaging it in a smaller battle that is sure to win. Moreover, some scientists argue that a low-dose exposure to ionizing radiation may in fact be healthful, and that it may prepare the cell for a subsequent high-dose exposure. For example,

> A-bomb survivors are living longer on the average than unexposed Japanese…. Nuclear shipyard workers

were much healthier than non-nuclear shipyard workers.... Areas with high natural background [radiation] have less cancer. (Cameron 1998)

Popularly referred to as radiation hormesis (Luckey 1991), this theory is not without its share of critics. Accepting that some but not all of the inevitable cell damage caused by ionizing radiation is soon repaired, and that it may even be beneficial, does not preclude the harsh reality that some damaged DNA can never be repaired:

There is *no* dose or dose-rate low enough to guarantee perfect repair of every carcinogenic injury induced by radiation. Some carcinogenic injuries are just unrepaired, unrepairable, or misrepaired. (Gofman 1990)

In a study of the effects of ionizing radiation on survivors of the 1945 atomic bombing of Hiroshima, the Radiation Effects Research Foundation concluded that there appears to be no low-dose threshold at which there is a zero risk of cancer (Pierce and Preston 2001).

Whatever the reality, the controversy rages between those who believe that there is a safe dose of ionizing radiation and those who argue otherwise. Either way, it is certainly not clear what constitutes a therapeutically safe dose of radiation—if indeed there is such a thing.

Radiography

X-rays were discovered accidentally in 1895 by the German physicist Wilhelm Conrad Röntgen (also spelled Roentgen). The well-known photograph of his wife's ring-fingered left hand is probably the first X-ray image of a living thing and marks the beginning of radiography. In 1913, the American physicist, William D. Coolidge invented the X-ray tube thereby making X-rays readily available for use in technology.

Radiography is photography that uses X-rays to produce a conventional emulsion film image. The familiar diagnostic photograph of radiopaque materials, such as bone, teeth, and dental fillings, is called an X-ray. Opacity is a measure of photon absorption and is proportional to the density of the irradiated tissue—bone is more opaque than muscle, muscle more opaque than fat, fat more opaque than fluid, and fluid more opaque than a void, such as an air pocket. The X-ray contrast of the less opaque bodily organs is sometimes temporarily improved by introducing a chemical agent to the person's biology.

Several examples are worth mentioning. A pyelogram is an X-ray picture of the urinary tract that is produced by intravenously (injected into a vein) introducing a radiopaque dye that concentrates in the urine and highlights the urinary vessels that are being irradiated. A cholecystogram is an X-ray picture of the gallbladder that is produced by having the patient ingest a contrast medium the night before examination. A barium enema is a procedure wherein a radiopaque solution is injected into the patient's rectum a few minutes before X-rays are taken of the large intestine thereby outlining the organ interior.

Other radiographic tools used in the cancer business include mammography, tomography, interventional radiology, and nuclear medicine.

Diagnostic X-Rays

An X-ray tube, in its simplest form, is a metallic and/or glass container housing a filament made of coiled tungsten wire, as that commonly found in an incandescent light bulb, and an anode made of tungsten or molybdenum or some other extremely high melting point heavy-element target all under vacuum (a very low pressure condition where gases have been removed). The filament is heated to an extremely high-temperature and electrons are accelerated to the anode by applying a voltage—the force that causes electricity to move–in this way generating X-rays at the anode surface. These relatively low-energy X-rays are transmitted out of the tube through a transparent window made of beryllium, a light-element with a relatively high melting point, for diagnostic purposes such as mammography.

Diagnostic X-rays typically have energies of 3 to 20 thousand electron volts (keV). Photons with this energy penetrate tissue and effect ionization to a depth of approximately 1 inch. An electron volt (eV) is equivalent to the energy an electron acquires while moving through a gradient of 1 volt (unit of voltage). And although higher voltages create higher-energy–more penetrating X-rays–it should be remembered that all X-rays are deadly, because all X-rays are capable of producing ionization. In fact, it was a mere 9 years after Röntgen's revolutionary discovery that the first human died as a result of exposure to this X-radiation, a name synonymous with X-rays.

People, however, are often slow to heed nature's warnings, and those responsible for our safety sometimes fail to protect us.   Some 7 years before the U.S. government alert of January 31, 2005, an unsuspecting public was warned that

> X-rays are carcinogenic. The more X-rays you submit to and the greater the dose, the greater is your risk of cancer. Avoid unnecessary X-rays like the plague.... Very few circumstances, if any, should persuade you to have X-rays taken if you are pregnant. (Epstein 1998, 304)

But not everyone hears, and even fewer listen. Diagnostic X-rays are all too commonly prescribed; this artificially produced radiation accounts for about 14% of the world's total exposure to X-rays. In the United States, diagnostic X-rays cause an estimated 5695 new cases of cancer per year, and roughly 0.9% of all cancer deaths. It is probably no coincidence that Japan, a country enamored with technology, has the highest number of new cancer cases linked to diagnostic X-rays in the world, since Japan uses diagnostic X-ray tubes more than any other country in the world (Berrington de Gonzalez and Darby 2004).

The danger of being exposed to artificial radiation is serious enough that the seemingly innocuous dental X-rays that many of us have experienced again and again are taken with most of our body protected by a heavy lead blanket and the technician or dentist standing in another room. Even then there is sufficient radiation leakage to cause low-term birth weight in women who unwittingly risked having a single dental X-ray taken while they were pregnant (Hujoel et al. 2004).

There is no doubt that diagnostic X-rays are extremely beneficial, and that X-ray tubes are essential in many applications. These include medicine, dentistry, materials inspection and analysis, cargo and baggage screening, and research and development, among other things. Indeed, X-ray tubes are ubiquitous and are manufactured by multi-national corporations—General Electric in the United States, Philips in the Netherlands, Siemens in Germany, and Toshiba in Japan. The largest wholesale supplier of X-ray tubes in the world is Varian Medical Systems, with its major X-ray tube manufacturing facility in Salt Lake City, Utah. Varian received more than $200 million in orders for 2005. X-ray tube technology is conceptually simple and mature in an engineering sense and is far from ever becoming obsolete.

Mammography

Mammograms are contrast-based film images that utilize diagnostic X-ray tubes to detect abnormalities often associated with breast cancer. In order to accommodate a low-energy X-ray, the breast must be severely flattened until it is thin enough for the beam of X-rays to pass through it and produce an acceptable photographic image of the internal anatomical structure. Low-dose radiation (typically 0.01 Gy per X-ray image) is necessary to minimize tissue damage and the associated inducement of cancer (Benke 1995). Mammograms are generally used to diagnose suspected cases of cancer in older women and to screen for cancer in young women who show no other symptoms of having the disease.

The Rochester, New York based Eastman Kodak Co. which accounts for more than half of the $1 billion worldwide X-ray film market, recently announced the availability of a film requiring half normal exposure time. Acknowledging the danger of mammograms, the company advertised:

> There are certainly health risks with exposure to radiation … there's universal agreement that less [radiation] is better. (Eastman Kodak Co. 2005)

Alternatively, a more costly digital X-ray imaging uses solid-state detectors, much like the familiar digital camera, to create a picture on a computer screen. This permits the radiologist (physician specialized in interpreting X-rays) to adjust the brightness and contrast, as well as to change the magnification of the image–alterations that are never without bias.

In early 2004, GE Healthcare, formerly GE Medical Systems, a $15 billion unit of General Electric headquartered in the U.K. and the leader in the digital mammography field, announced that it had installed 250 digital mammography systems worldwide, and that in less than 2 years it had imaged more than 1 million women in over 20 countries. By the end of 2005, GE claimed that it had installed over 1500 digital mammography systems worldwide.

Impressive for sure, but GE's digital imaging package has not reduced the dangerous X-ray exposure time, eliminated the painful and potentially harmful breast compression, or proved itself to be a better diagnostic tool than conventional film imaging. A University of North Carolina at Chapel Hill research study by Pisano and coworkers of 49,528 women in the United States and Canada concluded that the overall diagnostic accuracy of digital and film mammography as a means of screening for breast cancer is similar, but digital mammography is more accurate in women under the age of 50 years, women with radiographically dense breasts, and premenopausal or perimenopausal women. (Pisano et al. 2005)

This study failed to suggest a benefit for older women, whose breasts are generally less dense than those of young women and who account for more than half of the participants (Crystal and Strano 2006) that are most likely to develop breast cancer. Furthermore, the study suffers in that it is based on the interpretation of but two radiologists. The diagnosis (identification by its symptoms) of breast cancer via both digital and film mammography remains a highly specialized branch of medicine, and one that is all too subjective (Elmore et al. 1994): images of muscle, fat, and fluid appear as shades of gray against a black background, which according to Kopans, Halpern, and Hulka (1994) of the Harvard Medical School and Kerlikowske and coworkers (1998) of the University of California, San Francisco makes interpretation biased.

Screening–the detection of disease in the absence of cancer symptoms–is even a more difficult task. Using mammography for screening poses problems, one of which is that false-positive (mistakenly identified as cancer) mammograms are frequently observed in obese women, especially those with excess fatty breast tissue (Elmore et al. 2004). This is of growing concern in the United States in particular, where nearly 50 million American adults, half of them female, are classified as obese (currently defined as overweight by 30% or more). Moreover, false positives have the dubious distinction of almost always necessitating a biopsy (surgical removal of a tiny bit of tissue for microscopic diagnosis) with the accompanying stress of waiting to hear the verdict.

Breast implants, a popular addition of millions of women, further complicate mammographic screening because most implants are silicone (silicon-oxygen-based polymer) filled with either saline (solution of salt in water) or silicone gel, both of which are more radiopaque than normal breast tissue. Thus breast implants make it difficult to detect small tumors in particular (Smalley 2003). In the United States, 291,350 breast implants were performed in 2005 alone (American Society of Plastic Surgeons 2006).

In spite of an impressive list of technical advances, mammography screening is still unable to detect the earliest developing cancers and is plagued by false negatives and false positives; screening also misses interval cancers, and is subject to overdiagnosis (Epstein, Bertell, and Seaman 2001; Michell 2003). Simply put, false negatives are missed cancers and interval cancers are cancers that develop between mammographic screenings. Overdiagnosis is the misinterpretation of intraductal carcinoma as malignant (from the Latin *malignans*, i.e., acting maliciously).

Intraductal carcinoma, also called DCIS or ductal carcinoma-in-situ is uncommon in men, but it is the most common type of noninvasive breast cancer in women. It is often associated with tiny deposits of calcium that show up as white spots on X-ray mammograms, an artifact that further challenges the radiologist. DCIS is one of the few almost always-curable adenocarcinomas (cancers that originate in glandular tissue), provided that it has not spread past the milk ducts. The very term *in situ* means original position or place.

A number of scientists are quick to point out that patient mortality is not necessarily improved by early detection, and in fact, overdiagnosis of DCIS, benign tumors, and other false positives has lead to a disturbing 20% to 30% increase in unwarranted breast surgery (Olsen and Gotzsche 2001).

There is considerable debate over the age at which mammographic screening should begin. The American Cancer Society, the National Cancer Institute, the American Medical Association, and the American College of Radiology, as well as dozens more medical specialty organizations, claim a lower incidence of breast cancer mortality in women 40 years and older who undergo screening; whereas the American College of Physicians, the U.S. Preventive Services Task Force, and the Canadian Task Force on Preventative Health Care argue that screening should begin at age 50 years (Fletcher 1997).

Why all the controversy?

Premenopausal (time of life when menstruation is ongoing) women tend to have dense breast tissue that makes detection by mammography less reliable. Dense tissue and malignant tissue both appear white on an X-ray image making them indistinguishable. Moreover, since the low-dose exposure to X-rays inherent to mammograms is associated with an increased risk of cancer, younger women are actually advised to wait 5 to 10 years past the age when the U.S. government recommends that women receive their first mammogram (Brenner et al. 2002). Indeed, it has been suggested that only one life would be saved for every 1000 women aged 40 to 49 years old who were annually screened for 10 years and diagnosed for early breast cancer (Mokbel 2001). There is no debate that postmenopausal women benefit from screening:

> Most clinicians and researchers: agree that for women older than age 50 years, mammogram screening every 1-2 years reduces breast cancer deaths by 30%. For women younger than fifty, the efficacy of mammography in reducing cancer deaths has in past years been the subject of considerable debate. (McTiernan 2002)

The case for screening women more selectively and perhaps at later ages is supported by two facts. First, the rate of detecting breast cancer by mammography increases with age. Second, the incidence of breast cancer is generally higher in women having a first-degree relative—mother, daughter, or sister—who have already developed breast cancer (Kerlikowske et al. 2000).

The more frequently younger women undergo mammographic screening, the greater their total lifetime exposure to radiation with its associated risk of developing cancer. There is no scientific evidence to suggest a magic age at which mammography becomes beneficial. It is no surprise, then, that the age at which the National Cancer Institute recommends mammographic screening appears to be based more on politics than on science. Certainly the pressures of the financially lucrative mammography business are easy to understand. One prominent British specialist in breast cancer surgery puts it like this:

> The U.S. has the highest mastectomy rate worldwide.... The National Cancer Institute (NCI) appointed an independent panel which reviewed the available evidence and advised against screening women under age 50. But they were threatened that their budget would not be renewed unless they changed their tune.... Screening brings about more surgery overall. In the U.K., one third of detected breast cancers are subject to mastectomy.... No one in their right mind, outside the U.S., would offer mammography screening to women under age 50.... I think it's time women wised up to the fact that they're being duped.... In the U.S., screening is a huge commercial industry. (Baum 2002)

Worse yet, according to the University of California, San Francisco, there is some indication that medical practitioners in the United States tend to require further testing after mammography, and to perform more surgical biopsies, than medical practitioners in the U.K., even though the rate of tumor detection is the same in both countries (Smith-Bindman et al. 2006). It appears that America's "litigious atmosphere" forces physicians to protect themselves from being sued for failing to treat. Pressure from industry further contributes to this overprescription of testing fueled by the extensive efforts of radiation equipment manufacturers to sell their goods.

So is mammography an effective tool in reducing patient mortality from breast cancer?

Tabar and coworkers (2001) claim that regular mammographic screening every 1 to 2 years has resulted in a 63% reduction in death from breast cancer in Sweden. Other researchers, notably Gotzsche and Olsen (2000) and Miller (2003), have found no significant reduction in Denmark and Germany, respectively.

> If women choose mammography screening, they should understand that their risk of dying in the next few years may not be reduced. (Miller 2003)

Nonetheless, and in spite of its flaws, mammography, both film-based and digital, offers some women a sense of security, which may explain why it is a $1 billion business worldwide (Theta Reports 2003). The most recent U.S. data reveals that over 70% of all women 40 years old and older have had at least one X-ray mammogram within the past 2 years with the progressively more educated women in all age groups more likely to have had a mammogram than those women with less education (Centers for Disease Control and Prevention 2006b). It is no surprise then that women with private medical insurance were also more likely than those without medical insurance or even those with government subsidized insurance to have undergone mammography (Meissner, Breen, and Yabroff 2003). And perhaps nowhere else in the world does less education translate into less wealth and less health care than in the United States.

Since 1998, all Medicare (U.S. government funded program of guaranteed health insurance for people 65 years and older and those younger with certain disabilities) eligible women in the United States have been entitled to receive one annual mammogram. But mammograms cost money and, as of 2004, 45.8 million Americans—16% of the population—were without any medical insurance (DeNavas-Walt, Proctor, and Lee 2005) and many were unable to afford one.

A study conducted at Duke University found that 76% of women with health insurance had mammograms compared to 45% of uninsured women, and that women with private health insurance were more than twice as likely as uninsured women to undergo mammography (Taylor, Van Scoyoc, and Hawley 2002). Aside from the discovery of a breast anomaly (lump or other change) during self or clinical breast examinations, the recommendation of a woman's healthcare provider appears to be the foremost reason why women get mammograms. A collaborative Duke University—National Cancer Institute study added that socioeconomic factors—age, education, income level, health behaviors, health insurance, and provider characteristics—also play an important role in determining who gets mammograms (Dominick et al. 2003).

A study that examined 133,549 women in Arkansas found that African American women were less likely to obtain mammograms than Caucasian American women, noting in particular, that African American women 65 years and older were unlikely to have ever had a mammogram (Jazieh and Buncher 2002). Table 3.1 shows that a majority of African Americans and a significant percentage of Hispanic Americans are not counted among the near 5.5

Table 3.1

Racial distribution of U.S. women who got mammograms
between 1996 and 2004

Race/Ethnicity	Population (%)	Mammograms (%)
Caucasian	75.1	69.5
Hispanic	12.5	7.3
African American	12.3	5.2
Asian/Pacific Islander	3.7	4.9
Native American	0.9	1.1

Source: U.S. Census Bureau (2003); National Cancer Institute (no date).
Note: 2.4% of people responding to the census gave two or more races and 12% of the women who had mammograms were identified as mixed, other, or unknown.

million mammograms recorded between 1996 and 2004 by the U.S. government.

According to the National Cancer Institute in Bethesda, Maryland, mammographic screening in the United States increased from 30% in 1987 to 68% in 1998, while the use of low-cost clinical breast examinations actually declined from 83% to 76% in women age 40 to 49 years (Meissner, Breen, and Yabroff 2003). This cannot simply be because mammography is a more reliable detector of lethal breast cancer for clinical breast examinations are able to identify about 60% of the same cancers detected as well as some of the cancers undetected with mammography according to the University of Washington and Fred Hutchinson Cancer Research Center (Weiss 2003). And no one seems to dispute that the simple breast self-examination, with all its inherent inconsistencies in implementation, does improve a woman's chances of survival.

Perhaps the heightened self-awareness and the sense of control of one's destiny that a self-examination provides is a factor for survival. It is certainly hard to argue that there is any reason not to perform a no-cost breast self-examination, or for a medical practitioner not to take the extra 5 minutes to perform a clinical exam, especially in light of the ever-increasing cost of health care in the United States and elsewhere. Instead of discouraging the use of clinical and breast self-examinations, U.S. health care providers might follow a recommendation from Canada: when low-cost screening is combined with a judicious implementation of mammography based on the woman's age and family history, there is a concomitant increase in survival (Baines and Miller 1997; Harvey et al. 1997).

Tomography

Computed axial tomography (CAT) scanning, also called computed tomography (CT) imaging, uses diagnostic X-rays to create cross-sectional images of the body organs on a computer screen. This technology was developed more than 30 years ago by an American, Allan M. Cormack, and an Englishman, Godfrey N. Hounsfield and is used today primarily to diagnose cancers of the abdomen and chest—lung, liver, and pancreas—and to detect vascular (relating to blood vessels) disease and injury of the liver, spleen, and kidneys. In some cases, contrast dyes, intravenously injected, taken orally, or introduced rectally via enema, highlight specific organs or tissue and improve imaging.

CT scans are photographic slices (nominally ¼ inch thick) of the body–just like thin slices of bread–which a computer then compiles into a three-dimensional image of the scanned volume. The process typically takes less than 30 minutes and besides serving as a diagnostic tool for cancer, CT scans provide information on staging (determining how advanced the disease is), treatment planning (modeling the size and location of the tumor), and health monitoring (evaluating the effect of the treatment).

Virtual colonoscopy, also called computed tomographic colongraphy, uses CT scans to examine the large intestine while the intestine is expanded with air from a rectally inserted tube. It is intended to replace traditional colonoscopy (examination with a fiberoptically-coupled camera lens), which requires sedation, as a cancer-screening tool.

Recent studies of virtual colonoscopy at the Medical University of South Carolina have not been promising. In these studies, the technique detected only 39% of the small lesions (abnormal structures) and 55% of the large ones that were detected by conventional colonoscopy. The authors of this study regretfully concluded that "computed tomographic colonography ... is not yet ready for widespread clinical application. Techniques and training need to be improved" (Cotton et al. 2004).

The U.S. Food and Drug Administration (FDA) emphasizes that there is no data supporting the use of CT scans for screening people without symptoms. Furthermore, the Rochester, Minnesota Mayo Clinic in association with the Duke University Medical Center in Durham, North Carolina found that there was no proof of any benefit to utilizing CT screening for lung cancer (Patz Jr., Swensen, and Herndon II 2004).

Not to be deterred, a Hoag Memorial Hospital Presbyterian physician in California began offering whole-body scanning in 2001 through CT Screening International. This privately held company claimed to help people with lung and colon cancer and planned to open 300 centers in the United States alone (Finch 2002). At the end of 2002, CT Screening International shut down all of its centers leaving an answering machine to take calls and the FDA to account for its demise (Kaiser 2003):

> The principal risk associated with the radiation dose resulting to a person from a CT procedure is the small

> possibility of developing a radiation-induced cancer some time later in that person's life. (Food and Drug Administration 2005)

Nonetheless, the use of this relatively high-dose radiation procedure is actually increasing. Many medical researchers still claim that spiral CT screening (a modification by which the X-ray tube rotates around the patient and takes nonstop images as the patient is moved through the machine) can be made more effective than mammography in the detection of breast cancer, and that it is also an effective tool for the early detection of lung cancer (Pastorino 2006). Not so coincidentally, perhaps, the major manufacturers of X-ray tubes—GE, Philips, Siemens, and Toshiba—are also the principal suppliers of CT scanners.

A whole-body, multiple-slice CT scan exposes the patient to approximately 0.045 Gy. This is not an insignificant amount of radiation, given the Health Physics Society's warning to limit lifetime exposure to 0.01 Gy.

In the United States, CT scanning represents some 15% of all diagnostic radiology, and more than two-thirds of a person's lifetime total radiation dose (Wiest et al. 2002; Mettler Jr. et al. 2000). Similarly, in the U.K., one group found that CT scanning contributes to 40% of the total medical dose of all X-ray examinations (Shrimpton and Edyvean 1998).

The evidence suggests that being exposed to CT scans actually induces cancer, as the radiation dose from the CT scan is the same as the dose shown to be associated with an increased cancer risk in the survivors of the Hiroshima and Nagasaki atomic bombings (Brenner 2002). In the U.S. alone, if every smoker were given just one CT scan, the CT radiation risk could result in an additional 36,000 cases of lung cancer (Brenner 2004).

Even more disturbing is the fact that in the United States, some 6% of CT scans are performed on children (Brenner et al. 2001). Children are especially susceptible to radiation-induced cancers, because their smaller bodies receive a higher radiation dose per organ than adult bodies, their cells are more actively dividing, and they have more time to ultimately develop cancer (Brenner 2002). The National Cancer Institute (2002), reacting to the near 3 million annual CT examinations of children in the United States warns that "pediatric CT has become a public health concern."

Electron Beam Tomography (EBT) is an outgrowth of CT imaging used to screen for heart attacks (Gopal and Budoff 2006). Instead of mechanically rotating an X-ray tube around the patient, a precisely focused beam of electrons is electronically scanned around a tungsten target to produce a beam of X-rays that are rotated to provide scans in a fraction of a second. In spite of being able to create images that can freeze a beating heart, the patient is still exposed to a significant 0.0024 Gy (Leber et al. 2003) —a dose that is more than half the average annual background radiation.

Interventional Radiology

Diagnostic X-rays are a mainstay of image guidance procedures such as angiography (imaging blood vessels). Catheter angiograms are high-contrast X-ray images of arteries (arteriograms) and veins (venograms) produced by intravenously introducing a strongly absorbing X-ray-sensitive dye directly into the artery. Taking as long as 3 hours to complete, angiograms are used to evaluate peptic ulcers (sores in the stomach and/or small intestine); to diagnose diseases in the lung, brain, kidney, and blood-rich organs such as the liver; and to perform angioplasty, a nonsurgical procedure for opening clogged blood vessels.

The average radiation dose during angiography is approximately 0.006 Gy (Zanzonico, Rothenberg, and Strauss 2006).

It should be noted that angiograms are not always synonymous with X-rays. Fluoroscein angiography, for example, uses an intravenously injected sodium fluoroscein dye and ordinary photography to diagnose problems in the eye. Alternatively and sometimes in combination with the fluoroscein, indocyanine green dye is used as a marker if infrared photographic equipment is available.

A more advanced computerized form of X-ray angiography in which the radiopaque material is injected into a vein is called computed tomography angiography (CTA). According to the University of Chicago, CTA resembles CT scanning in that it allows for a three-dimensional anatomical reconstruction. This proves useful in diagnosing pulmonary embolisms (obstructions in the arteries of the lung), in assessing aneurysms of the aorta (balloon-like widening of the body's largest artery), and in evaluating potential kidney donors (MacEneaney and Dachman 2000). One obvious concern is that high-resolution images require more scans and a concomitant increase in X-ray exposure.

Other applications of interventional radiology include X-ray guided biopsy and accurately targeting the disease during cryosurgery (killing a tumor by repeatedly freezing and thawing it) and radioablation (killing a tumor by cooking it with internally administered radio frequency waves). X-ray imaging is also used during stenting, the placement of a tubular metal insert to open and support a blood vessel wall (angioplasty) or a biliary or other duct.

Nuclear Medicine

Radioactivity–the spontaneous emission of radiation–was first observed in 1896 by the Frenchman Antoine

Henry Becquerel in naturally occurring uranium, a chemical element. There are some 100 elements and approximately 2300 so-called isotopes (from the Greek *iso topos*, equal place) most of which are radioactive. An isotope is an element whose atoms have an equal number of protons and electrons, but a different number of neutrons.

Most naturally occurring elements, such as sodium and phosphorus, are stable. Some, however, such as uranium are only radioactive, and others, such as carbon and potassium may or may not be radioactive depending on what isotope is present. Radioactive isotopes are also called radioisotopes or radionuclides.

Isotopes are sometimes identified with a number suffix that defines the number of protons and neutrons. Uranium-238, used to fuel nuclear fission reactors; carbon-14, used to date ancient organic materials; and potassium-40, which is present in soil, sea water, and virtually all living organisms, are all naturally occurring radioisotopes. No naturally occurring radioisotopes are used to diagnose or treat cancer, whereas artificially made ones, first created by Frédéric and Irène Joliot-Curie in 1934, are the basis of nuclear medicine. Eight years after the Curies, Enrico Fermi and Leó Szilárd demonstrated the nuclear reactor, a device for the controlled splitting (fission) of a heavy atom. Today, many of the artificially produced radioisotopes used to treat cancer, such as phosphorus-32 and yttrium-90, are a product of the nuclear fission reaction.

All radioisotopes are characteristically unstable and spontaneously decay at a rate quantified by their half-life—the time required for their radioactivity to decrease by one-half. Thus, after one half-life, the radioactivity of a radioisotope is reduced by 50%; after two half-lives, by 25%; after three half-lives, by 12.5%; and so on. As the radioisotope decays, it is transformed into another element that may or may not be radioactive.

Some radioisotopes emit so-called beta radiation to achieve nuclear stability. Beta radiation is positively or negatively charged atomic particles called electrons, which are light, fast moving and capable of penetrating human tissue to a depth of 0.1 inch or so. Beta particles are as effective as X-rays in promoting ionization.

Other radioisotopes produce so-called alpha radiation when they disintegrate. Alpha radiation are helium nuclei— two protons and two neutrons—slow moving particles, very directional and are very readily absorbed in human tissue, but only penetrating a few cell diameters. Alpha particles have 20 times the ionizing power of X-rays and gamma rays, and because of their limited range, they dissipate all their energy within a cell or two, thus accounting for their deadliness. Unlike X-rays and gamma rays, there is no argument that a safe dose exists for alpha radiation and especially when it is inside the body.

And yet alpha rays are everywhere. Radon-222, a colorless, odorless, and tasteless gas that emits alpha particles and has a half-life of 3.82 days, is a natural decay product of the uranium-238 that is present in most soil. As such it contributes to the natural background radiation.

The nuclear transformation immediately following radioactive decay, in some cases, produces gamma radiation. Discovered by the French physicist Paul Villard in 1898, gamma rays are identical in all aspects to X-rays of equivalent energy except source. They penetrate human tissue just as deeply, and the damage to the cell is in all respects the same.

A number of elements, termed *metastable*, do not transform to another element at all when they decay–they simply emit gamma rays as a way of releasing their excess energy. The energy range of this decay scheme varies from 10 keV or so to several million electron volts (MeV). High-energy gamma emitters, such as technetium-99m (140 keV), have therapeutic value. In addition, there are a number of radioisotopes that emit low keV X-rays so that if nothing else, demonstrating that radioisotope radiation is diverse.

Like people, some elements are more interesting than others. All 22 technetium isotopes, for example, are radioactive, but only the metastable technetium-99m with its 6-hour half-life is widely used. In fact, it is by far the most commonly used radioisotope in diagnostic nuclear medicine. Created in a nuclear reactor, technetium-99m is used mostly as a radioactive tracer to image heart and skeletal tissue, the liver, the spleen, and in breast cancer patients, the lymph nodes (glands that fight infection).

Approximately 85% of all diagnostic nuclear medicine uses technetium-99m according to the Brookhaven National Laboratory on Long Island, New York (no date). The National Research Council of Canada (2003) adds that each week more than 100,000 people worldwide benefit from cancer treatment using technetium created in Canada. Pretty impressive considering that technetium, the first artificially produced element, did not even exist prior to 1937.

Another radioisotope commonly used in nuclear medicine is gallium-67, a liquid metal, low-energy (93 keV) gamma emitter with a relatively short 78-hour half-life. Gallium-67 is used to image inflammatory lesions in the lung and is produced in a cyclotron. This device was invented in 1929 by Ernest O. Lawrence to accelerate charged particles—alpha particles, protons and electrons—in a ring shaped vacuum chamber.

Beta-emitting radioisotopes like oxygen-15 and fluorine-18, also created with a cyclotron, are special in that they decay in the body to combine with a nearby electron and produce a gamma emission that may be subsequently located with a gamma radiation-sensitive camera. These gaseous radioisotopes can be taken intravenously or orally when tagged to a suitable molecule, or alternatively, introduced by inhalation for use as tracers in positron emission tomography (PET).   PET equipment is manufactured by Philips Medical Systems, GE Healthcare Bio-Sciences, Hitachi Medical Systems America Inc., and Gamma Medica-Ideas, Inc. (GMI) and used to detect cancer by identifying groupings of cells that are reproducing more rapidly than normal cells.

In single photon emission computed tomography (SPECT), a gamma-emitting radioisotope (e.g., technetium-99, iodine-123, or indium-111) is injected into the bloodstream to produce a three-dimensional digital image of the blood flow to the brain, heart, kidneys, and bone. This procedure is extremely controversial because the entire body is irradiated. SPECT equipment is supplied by Siemens Medical Solutions USA, Inc. and also GMI, the joint California-Norway business venture. SPECT warrants mentioning here only to illustrate how far some members of the medical and business community will go in the name of helping us to live a better life.

Kill or Be Killed

The idea of using deadly ionizing radiation as therapy is a bit of an oxymoron. High-dose radiation certainly does not heal and nor does it selectively kill only malignant cells—it kills all cells or at least disrupts the DNA in all cells that it contacts. In that sense, it is really no different than a surgeon's knife. Being bloodless makes it seem the much more friendlier killer.

The therapeutic value of radiation rests in its presumed ability to destroy a significantly greater number of bad cells than good ones, and not encourage any healthy cells to later become cancerous cells. The goal of treatment is to remove permanently all the cancer. Surgery is by far the most common method of treating cancer, and radiation is one highly sought after alternative.

Radiation Therapy

Various high-energy X-ray and gamma ray sources are used to treat cancer. Artificially produced X-rays are far and away the most frequently used form of radiation today and the technology for producing them is well developed. High-energy X-ray beams are mostly created using a linear accelerator, also called a linac. These rather large machines first produce very high-energy electrons that on passing through a thin tungsten target generate a beam of X-rays that are capable of penetrating human tissue to a depth of at least 6 inches thereby affecting ionization in any cell in the body.

In 1953, an 8 million volt (MV) linac was first used to treat English cancer patients in the U.K. Today, medical linacs operate from 5 MV to greater than 25 MV and are the workhorse of most modern cancer radiotherapy equipment collectively referred to as external beam radiation therapy (EBRT). Nothing else can so reliably deliver a deeply penetrating and deadly beam of radiation as linac based EBRT.

"We live and die by radiation therapy," touts the world's leading manufacturer of integrated cancer therapy systems with a near 60% of the world's oncology radiation market (Varian Medical Systems 2004a). Indeed, the Palo Alto, California based corporation has a near monopoly on radiotherapy equipment having sold more than 3500 linac based EBRT systems used to treat more than 1 million patients per year and over 50% of all cancer patients in the United States alone.

The Varian machines are extremely robust and dependable and have the advantage of producing a high energy X-ray beam only when the machine is turned on. As with most anything that is exposed to radiation, the irradiated parts of the machine become mildly radioactive thereby requiring safety and disposal considerations.

Instead of a machine with moving parts, a radioisotope alone can be used for radiotherapy. Cobalt-60, a gamma radiation source with a half-life of 5.27 years was first used in the U.K. by the London Regional Cancer Centre to treat cancer in 1951. The treatment was simple—expose the patient and the tumor to the stationary radiation source and let the deadly dual 1.17 and 1.33 MeV beam irradiate its human target.

The downside of these cobalt-60 machines is that the radiation source is always "turned on" and several inches of lead are required to protect everyone else from exposure (e.g., 2 inches of lead absorb 95% of a 1.5 MeV gamma ray beam). No less deadly than the manually on-off linac, this order of magnitude lower incident radiant energy only means less tissue penetrating power.

Today, MDS Nordion, the 8000 plus employee "global leader in radioisotope technology" with its main facility in Ottawa, Canada supplies more than 80% of the world's need for cobalt-60. The present day's version of the original cobalt-60 shuttered lead box is called a Gamma Knife, a far more sophisticated tool that features 201 digitally-focused gamma ray beams capable of delivering precise tumor targeting. This tool was invented in Sweden in 1968 by Lars Leksell a physician and is often referred to as the Leksell Gamma Knife in his honor.

Conformal Radiotherapy

Like a surgeon's scalpel, the radiation beam is imperfect in limiting its cutting edge to just the tumor. One of the major problems with EBRT is its inability to confine the lethal radiation to the malignancy so to avoid destroying healthy tissue. This problem is exacerbated in practice as the patient breathes and moves while being irradiated. Surprising no parent for sure, Fortney and coworkers (1999) report from the Duke University Medical Center that more than 93% of all children 2 years and younger require anesthesia during the most mundane radiation treatment to keep them immobile.

Intensity modulated radiation therapy (IMRT) uses highly sophisticated computer programs to *a priori* shape the radiation beam using a dynamic (time-dependent) computer model of the tumor (Bogardus 2000; Webb 2003). The idea here is to minimize the ratio of normal tissue dose to tumor dose. Conformality and pencil-tip accuracy of the radiation and at an elevated radiation dose are achieved. But to be truly effective, IMRT requires real time anatomical mapping of the target area during treatment to account for tumor movement, losses in tumor volume, and changes in the shape of the tumor. None of this can be modeled in real time with a computer and the medical practitioner must rely on such modeling to estimate the tumor's true location (Paliwal, Brezovich, and Hendee 2004).

And while the University of Chicago's Department of Radiation and Cellular Oncology suggests that IMRT is more useful to academic research than to patient therapy (Mell, Roeske, and Mundt 2003) there are other issues. Hall and Wu of the Columbia University College of Physicians and Surgeons (2003) and others (Bakai, Alber, Nusslin (2003) point out that the very nature of IMRT necessitates a longer radiation time, a larger volume of non-malignant tissue exposed to radiation, and an increase in total exposure—all of which nearly double the risk of radiation-induced secondary cancers with post-exposure lifetime:

> Whenever large-scale studies have been performed, radiotherapy has been showed to be associated with a statistically significant, although very limited increase in the risk of secondary malignancies particularly in long-term survivors. (Grégoire and Maingon 2004)

Aside from these drawbacks, the University of Wisconsin, Madison determined other reasons why only 10% of all radiotherapy patients actually benefit from IMRT. First, half of all patients who undergo radiotherapy are treated solely for palliation—pain relief—and palliation rarely requires pinpoint accuracy. Second, only 20% of the patients who do benefit—primarily those with tumors of the head, neck, and prostate—require IMRT's accuracy (Paliwal, Brezovich and Hendee 2004).

These realities, however, do not dissuade the companies with an investment in this technology:

> This is the most rapid adoption of a new form of radiotherapy that I have seen in my more than three decades of experience in radiation oncology ... with new reimbursement rates for IMRT, continuing product enhancements, better training, additional published clinical experience, and greater patient awareness, the pace of IMRT adoption is likely to remain rapid ... the amount of research into its potential has exploded. (Varian Medical Systems 2002)

Varian Medical Systems is the world's largest seller of IMRT systems, out-selling Siemens, the multinational conglomerate headquartered in Germany that employs some 400,000 people worldwide, and two smaller corporations, Elekta, Inc. in Sweden, and North American Scientific in the United States combined. IMRT has been good to Varian business and its 2006 stock price had increased ten-fold since 1999. Varian Medical Systems had even outperformed the Dow, the Nasdaq, and the S&P by more than 500% making IMRT very profitable:

> IMRT can be a very lucrative addition to both freestanding centers hospital based radiation oncology programs. The procedure's profit comes from the fee for technical services (around $400 per treatment) compared to around $100 per treatment for conventional radiation oncology. (Bogardus Jr. 2003a)

Why is IMRT so expensive?

The physicist, the dosimetrist, and the radiation oncologist must devote almost three times the amount of planning time to an IMRT case than is required for either conventional external beam or 3D-CRT therapy. (Bogardus Jr. 2003b)

The high cost of IMRT is in part why in the United States Medicare reimburses hospitals for IMRT at a higher rate than conventional radiotherapy. Hospitals are in fact encouraged to implement IMRT despite there being no randomized clinical trial data supporting its widespread use (Guerrero Urbano and Nutting 2004; Hong et al. 2005).

On October 20, 2004, Varian Medical Systems and GE Healthcare announced yet another improvement in radiotherapy. The two giants combined GE's PET scan– "captures the metabolic activity of the tumor" and CT scan– "provides high-resolution images clearly depicting the tumor's location and structure" with Varian's "respiratory gating" IMRT equipment:

Using these different technologies has enabled us to discover very unexpected movement in some of the tumors. If the patients had been treated conventionally, the tumors would have moved out of the treatment field and we might have under-treated them. (Holy Name Hospital 2004)

This not so reassuring endorsement of IMRT highlights the incredible difficulty of limiting a beam of ionizing radiation to only destroying cancerous tissue.

Stereotactic Radiosurgery

Seventeen years before the Gamma Knife, Lars Leksell, invented the concept of radiosurgery—a one-session radiation therapy. Radiosurgery uses precisely guided radiation from a linac or a Gamma Knife to destroy tumors. It is not surgery *per se* but a physically non-invasive treatment that requires no incision. Unlike traditional surgery, radiosurgery is not associated with complications due to infection, anesthesia side effects, facial weakness, hearing loss, and brain stem injury (Rosenberg, Zerris, and Borden 2001). When radiosurgery is coupled with stereotactic placement in which the head and neck are physically fixed during treatment via a three-dimensional skeletal positioning device, the accuracy of radiosurgery is improved and higher-doses are realized.

According to American Shared Hospital Services (AMS), a 12-person publicly traded company based in San Francisco providing Gamma Knife support to hospitals in the United States there are approximately 103 Gamma Knife centers in the United States and 234 units installed worldwide as of 2006. AMS claims that each center treats on average 175 patients annually. Elekta, Inc., the company that manufactures the Gamma Knife, reported in 2006 that more than 350,000 patients had been treated in more than 220 hospitals worldwide with their product.

Enhanced Radiotherapy

It is well established that tumor cells that have become hypoxic or oxygen deficient are the most resistant to radiation, requiring up to a three times higher radiation dose to destroy. These cancers are so resistant in fact that cancer patients with hypoxic tumors are sometimes asked to breathe a gas mixture containing less than half the oxygen by volume in air while being irradiated.

The air we breathe is normally 78% nitrogen, 21% oxygen, and less than 1% other gasses—argon and carbon dioxide—by volume. In hypoxic radiotherapy, the use of air with less oxygen momentarily renders nearby healthy tissue just as radiation resistant as the hypoxic tumor which then increases the selectivity of destroying malignant tumors over healthy tissue.   Alternatively, in hyperbaric radiotherapy, the patient is placed in a chamber with 100% oxygen at greater than one atmospheric pressure while being treated. This technique has been used in Europe by a working oncology group and reported as improving overall survival and local tumor control in head and neck cancers as well as in managing radiation-induced complications after irradiation (Mayer et al. 2005).

Hypoxic modifying drugs are also employed in combination with radiotherapy to improve tumor selectivity. Cisplatin, an organic-platinum compound approved for use in the United States by the Food and Drug Administration in 1978 for chemotherapy, is an example of a radiosensitizer—a drug that under certain conditions makes a cancer cell more sensitive to the effects of ionizing radiation.

Brachytherapy

Brachytherapy is a form of radiotherapy in which the radiation source is placed in direct contact with the cancer. This concept of internal radiotherapy was apparently first suggested in 1903 by Alexander Graham Bell—the inventor of the telephone using naturally occurring radium.

One of brachytherapy's earliest patients was the remarkable Giacomo Puccini.   In 1924, this perennial smoker of cigars was diagnosed with an incurable form of cancer of the larynx (voice box) and treated with both internal and external radium brachytherapy. Within 4 days of treatment Puccini's heart failed and the world lost the last great composer of opera (Marchese-Ragona, Marioni, and Staffieri 2004).

A wide variety of radioisotopes for use in brachytherapy are artificially produced in both nuclear reactors and in cyclotrons.   The Oak Ridge National Laboratory in Tennessee is a major source of reactor fission products in the United States. Smaller nuclear reactors are also used throughout the world to produce specific isotopes. Cyclotrons are more costly to operate than reactors but they have the advantage of producing radioisotopes with higher specific activities (amount of radioactivity per amount of material) and radioisotopes that are free of other radioisotopes.

Brachytherapy has evolved into a relatively small cancer therapy business. The sale of all brachytherapeutic products in the United States was $321 million in 2002 and projected to grow to $1.3 billion in 2008. Nucletron, a subsidiary of Delft Instruments N.V. is a publicly traded Dutch medical device company specializing in brachytherapy cancer treatment. Established in 1975, the company reported a net profit of $13 million in 2002.

In high-dose rate (HDR) brachytherapy, a wire tipped with a gamma-emitting radioisotope is inserted in a catheter (a slender flexible tube) that has been placed inside a tumor (called an interstitial implant procedure) or near a tumor. The radioactive source is positioned in the tumor for a relatively short period of time. This treatment has been applied to cancers of the prostate, esophagus, lung, and breast, among others. Intracavity brachytherapy, for example, is used to treat cervical and vaginal cancers by temporarily holding a radioactive source inside the vagina. Iridium-192, a gamma emitter with an average energy of 400 keV and a 74-day half-life is the radioisotope used in the HDR equipment manufactured by both Nucletron and Varian Medical Systems.

Alternatively, in early stages of prostate cancer, dozens of lower-dose radioactive seeds–metal encased radioisotopes the size of a grain of rice–are surgically implanted directly into the tumor to remain and radiate according to their half-life. In both cases, healthy tissue is damaged in so far as to the extent that it is affected by the attenuated radiation source. Radiation dissipates inversely as the distance from the source is squared—tissue twice as far away from the radioactive seed receives ¼ the dose.

Iodine-125 (60-day half-life) and palladium-103 (17-day half-life) are the two most commonly used radioisotopes in permanent seed implants. These isotopes are a source of 27 keV gamma rays and 21 keV X-rays, respectively and thus afford the clinician relatively easy protection because of their low energy.

Radioactive gold-198 (combination gamma plus beta emitter with a 2.7-day half-life) is another attractive seed implant. Gold is chemically inert and so as in dentistry, it finds use in the treatment of tongue cancer, a place in the body where most metals would corrode and ultimately dissolve in the saliva (spit) and plaque bacteria mix (Kimura et al. 2003). Moreover, because gold is extremely radiopaque it is also an excellent marker for CT scans.

Permanent seed implants can affect lifestyle. In one case at least, a cancer patient undergoing permanent seed implant treatment was sufficiently radioactive to have set-off an airport security alarm (WorldNetDaily.com 2004). More generally, the practice of safe sex, even with a condom, and the sitting of a grandchild on the lap is problematic.

Radioimmunotherapy

Immunotherapy describes treatment that is intended to restore the ability of the body to fight infection. When combined with radiation this treatment is referred to as radioimmunotherapy (RIT). In this method, alpha or beta emitting radioisotope tagged monoclonal antibodies (MAbs) —laboratory synthesized proteins that preferentially attach themselves to tumor cells and signal the body's immune cells to respond favorably—are used to target specific disease sites minimizing toxicity to normal cells (Rao, Akabani, and Rizzieri 2005, of the Duke University Medical

Center in North Carolina; Burke, Jurcic, and Scheinberg 2002, of the Memorial Sloan-Kettering Cancer Center in New York City).

RIT is expensive, each dose costing several tens of thousands of dollars because of the difficulty of incorporating a radioactive element in a complex organic molecule. Unlike all other radiation based therapies, RIT doses are usually expressed in milliCurie (mCi) units, which are a measure of the rate and not the energy of the radiation emitted from a radioisotope.

Iodine-131, a combination beta plus gamma emitter with an 8-day half-life was approved for RIT in the United States by the Food and Drug Administration (FDA) in June 2003. Its gamma radiation allows for external detection and calculation of the ratio of tumor dose to normal tissue dose, but necessitates

> maintaining a safe distance of at least 6 feet, when possible from others (particularly children and pregnant or nursing mothers), abstaining from intercourse, using a separate bathroom, bagging all clothing and washing them separately from other members of the family, using a separate set of dishware and washing it separately, eliminating wastes while sitting at all times and flushing at least 2 times with the seat down and throwing away the toothbrush used after 2 weeks. (Rao, Akabani, and Rizzieri 2005)

Yttrium-90, a pure 2.28 MeV beta emitter approved for RIT by the FDA in February 2002, is safer to use than iodine-131 and lends itself to outpatient (patent goes home the same day) treatment, but does not permit dosimetry. The dosimetry problem was addressed with some success by a Mayo Clinic researcher who added a gamma emitting indium-111 pretreatment to yttrium-90 RIT experimental cancer trials (Witzig 2004).

Alpha emitting actinium-225 (10-day half-life) and bismuth-213 (46-min half-life) labeled MAbs are being explored (Burke, Jurcic, and Scheinberg 2002) but no alpha radiation sources are as yet FDA approved. Alpha emitters are ideally suited for RIT because they deliver extremely high doses of lethal radiation in cellular distances and present no inordinate handling difficulties. Moreover, because their penetrating range is but a fraction of beta sources toxicity to normal cells is minimal.

Particle Radiation Therapy

In addition to alpha and beta particles, other kinds of subatomic particles can be used to kill cancer cells. Protons, first discovered in 1918 by Ernest Rutherford, the father of nuclear physics, are hydrogen ions—positively charged particles that are 1836 times heavier than electrons. In an uncharged atom, the number of protons always equals the number of electrons. Protons if accelerated to a high velocity easily penetrate human tissue and deposit their maximum energy at a depth that is proportional to the accelerating voltage. The maximum energy has a bell-shaped distribution (called a Bragg peak) that can be concentrated in the tumor and so unlike photons that continue to propagate unless annihilated, the collimated or focused proton beam is even more conformal than IMRT. Like high-energy photons, protons ionize atoms and consequently damage DNA. High-energy protons are therapeutically attractive in that they are five times as effective as equivalent energy photons in causing permanent cellular damage.

Proton therapy was first used to treat cancer in 1954. Treatment is not readily accessible, however, because proton therapy facilities cost $100 to $200 million and take several years to build. In fact, there are less than two-dozen proton therapy facilities in the world with no more than 45,000 people treated to date. Proton therapy first became available in the United States in 1990 at the Loma Linda University Medical Center in California. Since then 50 tumor types in some 12,000 patients have been treated at Loma Linda (National Association for Proton Therapy 2006). Other proton treatment facilities in the United States include the Francis H. Burr Proton Therapy Center, Massachusetts General Hospital, Boston; the Midwest Proton Radiotherapy Institute at Indiana University, Bloomington; the Texas M. D. Anderson Proton Therapy Center; and the University of Florida's Shands Medical Center in Jacksonville, Florida.

Fourteen years after Rutherford's remarkable discovery, James Chadwick in the U.K. identified another deadly radiation product—the neutron. Energetic neutrons are uncharged particles that are slightly heavier than protons and also of therapeutic value because when they quite literally collide with water molecules inside the cell they ionize the surrounding tissue. High-energy neutrons are needed to cause permanent tumor damage and so huge accelerators are required to produce them. The availability of this costly and highly specialized technology is even more limited than proton therapy. There are only three such facilities in the United States, none of which were originally built to treat cancer. Notwithstanding the lack of availability, the Fermilab in Illinois has treated more than 3000 cancer patients since 1976.

Alternatively, neutron brachytherapy (NBT) is also being explored using californium-252 (2.645-year half-life), an intense neutron emitter. This radioisotope is produced only in Russia, and at the Oak Ridge National Laboratory nuclear reactor in the United States. Although NBT has been investigated for several decades, it has only been used to treat a few-hundred cancer patients a year worldwide due to its limited availability (Martin and Miller 2002). And like its ionizing brethren, exposure to neutron radiation is also not without risk of developing cancer:

> Neutrons cause genetic damage similar to that caused by X-radiation and gamma radiation, and they also produce gamma radiation when they interact with biological materials and thus would cause the same cancers as X-radiation and gamma radiation. (National Institute of Environmental Health Sciences 2005b)

A Big Problem with Cancer

Heredity (passing of a trait from parent to offspring) or at least the shared environment inherent in familial relationships often harshly condemns some of us to develop cancer before birth (Heeg et al. 2006). Cancer has even caused death in the unborn according to the University of California, San Francisco (Jennings et al. 1993). Luckily, cancer is inherited no more than 5% of the time (Sifri, Gangadharappa, and Acheson 2004). A report from Iceland adds that the risk of developing cancer is significantly higher when genetics (science of how things pass down from parent to child to grandchild and so on) reveals that a close family member has been diagnosed with cancer; the exceptions being nonmelanoma skin, melanoma, and brain cancers (Amundadottir et al. 2004).

Size Matters

If a mutated cell divides too rapidly and its progeny ultimately develop into a massive collection of abnormal cells, the result is called a tumor. A tumor, also called a neoplasm, is a growth that has no physiological function, meaning it serves no useful purpose. Tumor cells are sometimes so prolific that they outgrow their blood supply and become hypoxic.

Tumors are benign (non-cancerous) if they remain localized in their place of origin and malignant if they spread to other parts of the body. Both types of tumor can be fatal because they stress bodily functions. It is important to understand that removal of a benign tumor is curative, whereas removal of a malignant one is not necessarily curative and may eventually result in death.

Tumors are often characterized by their size. Large tumors are in general a more serious health risk than smaller ones and so there is a need to communicate their relative size. The most commonly accepted system for describing tumor size defines a T1 tumor as one that is less than 1 inch in its greatest dimension. A T2 tumor is more than 1 inch but less than 2 inches in size and a T3 tumor is one greater than 2 inches in any one dimension.

Metastasis describes the spreading of malignant cells from a primary cancer site (place of origin) to another organ or tissue where they then become secondary tumors. Metastases (plural) proceeds via the circulatory system (heart, blood, and blood vessels) and the lymphatic system. An average adult has about 5 liters of blood accounting for about 8% of the body weight and three times as much lymph (fluid containing white blood cells and antibodies). It is therefore easy to understand that how a secondary tumor can develop quickly and appear almost anywhere in the body.   These secondary tumors have the same histology (microscopic structure) as those in the tumor of origin and in such a way can be used to identify the primary tumor site. Breast cancer that has metastasized to the lung, for example, appears as breast cells when examined microscopically. Often it is the metastasized tumor that is discovered first. However, identifying a cancer's origin is not straightforward. Each year in the United States

> several thousand people are diagnosed with metastatic cancer whose primary cancer site is not known. When the primary site cannot be identified, this disease may be called carcinoma of unknown primary (CUP). (National Cancer Institute 2004)

Eventually four out of five CUP are identified. In Greece, for example, CUP most frequently originate in the lung or pancreas with the liver being the primary metastatic site (Pavlidis et al. 2003). In Iraq, the most common metastatic site is the liver followed by bone (Hashim and Al-Quryni 2005). In Bahrain, a 50-plus year analysis showed a 4.5% CUP incidence; the most common metastatic site was the lymph nodes followed by the liver (Al-Hilli and Ansari 2005). Histology is art as well as science and so roughly 3% of CUP worldwide remain unidentified even following a post-mortem examination (National Cancer Institute 2005e).

In order to evaluate patient prognosis and begin treatment planning, the disease must be staged. Cancer staging is a method by which the primary tumor and its spread through out the body are quantified. Staging allows for a common language among the medical community so that various treatments can be compared. The TNM (Tumor, Node, Metastasis) staging system is based on a five level classification that evaluates the abnormality of the cancer cell, the size of the tumor, the tumor location, the organs that have been affected by the primary tumor, and the extent of metastasis if any that has occurred.

All stage 0 tumors are benign. Localized malignant tumors are termed stage I. Stage II malignancies are those that have spread beyond the primary tumor site to adjacent tissue. These malignancies include T2 and lower size tumors. Stage III malignancies have more aggressively invaded surrounding tissue. Stage III malignancies include T3 and lower size tumors. And finally, stage IV tumors are those cancers characterized with distant metastasis. Stage IV malignancies are the most deadly and may include any size primary tumor. In general, a higher staging number is associated with a more progressed disease and a worse prognosis. More often than not, early detection is the key to surviving cancer.

Roll the Dice

Once cancer is staged, prognosis, and treatment are often evaluated through clinical trials (use of volunteers to test new methods). These studies require delicately balancing survival and quality of life—the ever-elusive state of overall well-being and general sense of comfort (Greisinger et al. 1997; Janda et al. 2004). One of the tools cancer researchers employ to measure survival is statistics, a branch of mathematics concerned with the collection of numerical data for use in analyzing random events, such as the effect of a particular therapy on mortality.

Statistics can be deceiving and the conclusions that are derived from them are ideally based on randomized samplings (non-preselected patients) that are a key component as is a control (a like-sampling of patients not undergoing the same treatment). But randomness is not easily achieved because in general people do not seek treatment until after being evaluated and no health care provider willingly withholds treatment for the sake of science. Moreover, the sample selected is a function of socioeconomics and prone to erroneous conclusions that one sex, race or ethnic group is more inclined to develop or die from a particular cancer than another.

Instead of using crude (raw) data, statisticians frequently use age-adjustment (a process whereby differences in the age composition of two or more populations are removed). An aging population is expected to exhibit a year-to-year increase in mortality as its older members contribute more and more to the total number of deaths. When age-adjusted, the cause-specific mortality should in theory, show trends due to factors other than age. Age-adjustment is used only for comparison, as it does not reflect the true population, whereas the crude rate is a true measure of the actual incidence and is always higher than the age-adjusted rate.

Sometimes, so-called meta-analysis (combining results of two or more studies) is useful for developing a single conclusion by reevaluating the results of previously published randomized clinical trials. Controlled clinical trials more commonly use things like medical record numbers and patient social security numbers in the United States, neither of which are truly random. Irrespective of the real randomness of any study, a large sampling of cancer patients results in statistics that in general, more credibly reflect the larger real world population. The Massachusetts General Hospital in Boston and countless other facilities have emphasized that the reliability of the statistics used to evaluate the efficacy of cancer treatment must always be evaluated in terms of the bias of the statistician (Kopans, Halpern, and Hulka 1994).

Scientific objectivity can be difficult to achieve in practice especially when the researcher wants to do good or is faced with the prospect of drawing an unfavorable conclusion and losing funding. Intentional bias is often the result of pressure from those power brokers with vested interests who ultimately finance the research.

Epidemiology uses statistics to study incidence and mortality. The average is the mean and the median is the division of the sample into equal halves. Mortality is defined as death. Rates in the United States for some ethnic groups—notably American Indian and Pacific

Islanders—are often underestimated by as much as 20% and more according to Hoyert and Anderson (2001) of the National Cancer Institute. The cause-specific or disease-specific mortality is even more subjective than the total mortality in that it requires specifying a primary cause of death after a cancer patient may have experienced treatment related side effects any one of which could have been fatal. It may in fact not at all be apparent whether the cancer or the cancer treatment itself shortened the patient's survival. And metrics like disease-free survival (the length of time after treatment in which no cancer is found) are problematic as patients are lost during follow-up.

Morbidity (the incidence of a disease) is another important metric used in clinical trials. The difficulty with using morbidity as a measure of treatment success is that a particular therapy may in fact be 100% successful in curing the targeted disease, while at the same time introducing other complications or diseases that ultimately reduce the cancer patient's overall survival rate (percentage of people alive after treatment). This is especially true in the elderly, and in people with other ailments, or limited health care coverage.

Retrospective statistical studies are always undertaken many years after the first treatment. These studies are typically not done by the original investigators and are often used to uncover the true therapeutic response with a long-term view. Prospective studies, on the other hand, are designed by the original researchers who follow a treatment after it has been given and in so doing evaluate its effect. In certain cases, conclusions are actuarial—based on projections.

The bottom line is that both medical researchers and cancer patients desire concrete numbers, statistics to help guide decisions regarding the necessary trade-offs required to ensure a certain quality of life. Meaningful statistics that support such choices are often unavailable. So many clinical studies conclude with "additional research is needed," "deserve further investigation," and "warrant further evaluation"—statements that fail to comfort cancer patients, who no longer have the luxury of time.

Really Not Improving with Age

Cancer has been called a disease of aging. Almost 70% of the people who die from it are 60 years and older and 44% are over 70 years old (World Health Organization 2005a). The Memorial Sloan-Kettering Cancer Center in New York City states that persons 65 years and older have a roughly ten times higher incidence of cancer than younger people (Hurria and Kris 2003).

Table 5.1 compares the most recently available cancer incidence and disease-specific mortality in four industrialized countries. The divergence between crude

Table 5.1

Aging world population, estimated cancer incidence, and cancer mortality

	U.S.	Canada	Japan	U.K.
Population age 65 and older (%)	12.5	13.3	20.0	15.8
Incidence (cases per 100,000 population)	470 (431)	415 (447)	230 (415)	- (467)
Mortality (deaths per 100,000 population)	190 (192)	179 (207)	142 (243)	- (256)

Source: Jemal et al. (2006); National Cancer Institute (2006a); Canadian Cancer Society (2006); National Cancer Center (2005); Cancer Research UK (2002); U.S. Central Intelligence Agency (2006).
Note: Nonmelanoma skin cancers are excluded. Statistics are age-adjusted and (crude).

rates and age-adjusted rates is proportional to the percentage of how old the population. Crude rates show that Japan has fewer cases of cancer than the U.S., the U.K., and Canada, and when adjusting for age, Japan still has about half as many cases as Canada and the U.S. Age-adjusted rates also show that Japan has a lower death rate from cancer than Canada and the U.S., while the U.S. has the fewest cancer deaths overall.

While no one disputes that age is cancer's greatest risk factor, the prospect of eventually developing cancer is not simply just a part of life's programming and may rather be a result of a life-time accumulation of cellular trauma (Macieira-Coelho 2001). Cancer is in fact quite often a result of exposure to carcinogens.

A carcinogen is anything proved to cause cancer. Carcinogenicity (ability to cause cancer) is not always easy to establish. The element chromium, for example, is not carcinogenic unless its atoms are ionized such that they are missing six electrons (hexavalent chromium). If each atom is missing only three electrons (trivalent chromium) then chromium is not carcinogenic and is in fact essential for life. No one disputes that hexavalent chromium is a carcinogen when inhaled, but agreement on its carcinogenicity when ingested is still debated. In other words, the manner in which a material is introduced into the body is critical to its effect on the cells. Attempting to prove something is carcinogenic is difficult because it is not always easy to create a controlled environment with humans and even then susceptibility varies with stage of life (infancy, childhood, and adult).

Generalities help and in the United States, the Environmental Protection Agency (EPA) provides categories such as, "human carcinogen," "probable human carcinogen," possible human carcinogen," "not classifiable as to human carcinogenicity," and "likely to be carcinogenic to humans," to help Americans avoid the wrong stuff altogether (Environmental Protection Agency 1999). Another U.S. government agency, the National Institute for Occupational Safety and Health actually lists a number of "potential occupational carcinogens" but some of the culprits—asphalt fumes, diesel exhaust, environmental tobacco smoke, gasoline, nickel, silica, and wood dust—are so pervasive and unavoidable that the list does little more than contribute to an already paranoid lifestyle (Centers for Disease Control and Prevention 2004b).

Whether cancer is a birthright, a consequence of aging, a result of greater life-long exposure to carcinogens, or all three, there is no arguing that cancer is more common in older people.

Numbers Do Not Lie

Life is unfair and cancer is surely one reflection of its injustice. Lance Armstrong, the record setting *Tour de France* champion bicyclist, and Brian Piccolo, the football running-back depicted in the twice made movie *Brian's Song* are two Caucasian American athletes who both, at 25 years, were diagnosed with nonseminomas (a type of testicular cancer). The two men were subsequently treated with the world's best available surgical resection and chemotherapy. The hapless 26-year old Piccolo died in 1970 within one year of the discovery of a tumor in the center most part of his chest. Diagnosed in October 1996, the truly amazing Armstrong won his seventh consecutive *Tour* in 2005.

Maybe it is all a matter of luck. However, one thing is certain—the number of newly diagnosed cases of cancer and the deaths from cancer continues to increase annually throughout the world, including the United States and in proportion to the country's aging population, even when adjusted for age (table 5.2). Here, the number of cases of

Table 5.2

Cancer incidence and mortality in the United States

Year	Incidence (number of cases)	Mortality (number of deaths)
2006	1,399,790	564,830
2005	1,372,910	570,280
2004	1,368,030	563,700
2003	1,334,100	556,902
2002	1,284,900	557,271
2001	1,268,000	553,768
2000	1,220,100	553,091

Source: Jemal et al. 2002, 2003, 2004, 2005, 2006; Greenlee et al. 2000, 2001.

Note: Nonmelanoma skin cancers are excluded. Deaths are estimated after 2003 and age-adjusted to the 2000 U.S. population. 2002, 2001, and 2000 statistics are age-adjusted to the 1970, 1997, and 1996 U.S. population.

cancer reported annually reflects only those patients actually diagnosed with cancer and not those unwittingly stricken with the disease. Also, the number of cancer deaths in any particular year reflects an accumulation of all those people diagnosed, or never diagnosed, over a period of many years:

The drop in the actual number of cancer deaths in 2003 and in our own projections for 2006 mark a remarkable turn in our decades-long fight to eliminate cancer as a major health threat. For years, we've proudly pointed to dropping cancer death rates even as a growing and aging population meant more actual deaths. Now, for the first time, the advances we've made in prevention, early detection, and treatment are outpacing even the population factors that in some ways obscured that success. (American Cancer Society 2006a)

In spite of this optimism, the World Health Organization (2005b) laments that "only one-third of all cancers can be cured by earlier detection combined with effective treatment" because in truth, all cancers are not the same.

Certain tissues (collection of cells united in a particular function) and organs (group of tissues that perform a function) are more likely to be diagnosed as the primary site. Table 5.3 shows that in the United States, where there are 1.4 times as many women as men 65 years and older (U.S. Central Intelligence Agency 2006), cancer of the prostate gland is the most commonly identified cancer site in males, and cancer of the breast is the most frequently identified cancer site in females.

Table 5.3

Common site-specific cancers in the United States

Cancer	Cases (per year)	Deaths (per year)
Prostate	234,460	27,350
Breast	214,640	41,430
Lung and bronchus	174,470	162,460
Colon	106,680	55,170
Melanoma (skin)	62,190	7,910
Urinary bladder	61,420	13,060
Non-Hodgkin lymphoma	58,870	18,840
Rectum	41,930	55,170
Endometrium (uterus)	41,200	7,350
Kidney	38,890	12,840
Leukemia	35,370	22,280
Pancreas	33,730	32,300
Thyroid	30,180	1,500
Stomach	22,280	11,430
Ovary	20,180	15,310
Brain, nervous system	18,820	12,820
Liver	18,510	16,200
Multiple myeloma	16,570	11,310
Esophagus	14,550	13,770
Mouth	10,230	1,870
Cervix	9,710	3,700

Table 5.3 (Continued)

Cancer	Cases (per year)	Deaths (per year)
Soft tissue	9,530	3,500
Larynx	9,510	3,740
Tongue	9,040	1,780
Pharynx	8,950	2,110
Gallbladder	8,570	3,260
Testis	8,250	370
Hodgkin lymphoma	7,800	1,490
Small intestine	6,170	1,070
Anus	4,660	660
Vulva	3,740	880
Bone	2,760	1,260
Ureter	2,430	770
Vagina	2,420	820
Eye	2,360	230
Penis	1,530	280

Source: Jemal et al. (2006).

Note: Statistics are age-adjusted. Colon and rectum cancer deaths are combined. Soft tissue cancers include muscle, cartilage, tendon, fat, and not bone.

Table 5.3 also shows that some cancers are more lethal than others. Cancer of the lung and bronchus (tubular connection to the windpipe) is the third most common cancer in the United States and yet it kills more men and women than any other five types of cancer combined. Cancer of the colon is the fourth most often diagnosed U.S. cancer and when the number of deaths it causes is combined with that of cancer of the rectum— colorectal cancer is America's second deadliest cancer.

According to the National Cancer Institute (NCI), cancer treatment expenditure is aptly described as the sum of three phases: initial (diagnosis and therapy); continuing (surveillance and post-therapy); and terminal (palliation and hospice) (Brown et al. 2002). Cancers that lend themselves to screening (breast, colorectal, and prostate) tend to have the highest initial treatment costs. Cancers that are the least treatable (pancreas, lung, and esophagus) tend to have the lowest continuing costs. And cancers with the highest survival rates (prostate, bladder, and melanoma) tend to have the lowest terminal costs.

Cancer is a chronic disease. The total cost of cancer treatment in the United States is almost $75 billion per year (Reeder and Gordon 2006). Table 5.4 shows that while the most frequently diagnosed cancers are also the most costly cancers to treat; the money the NCI devotes to research is not commensurate with the cost of treatment.

Table 5.4

Federal money allocated annually for cancer
treatment and cancer research in the United States

Cancer	Treatment ($ million)	Research ($ million)
Lung	9,600	279.2
Colon and Rectum	8,400	262
Breast	8,100	570
Prostate	8,000	310
Lymphoma	4,600	118.4
Bladder	2,900	34.8
Leukemia	2,600	217.9
Ovary	2,200	100
Kidney	1,900	30.5
Endometrium	1,800	27.5
Cervix	1,700	79.0
Melanoma	1,500	102.9
Pancreas	1,500	53.7
Esophagus	779	21.9

Source: National Cancer Institute (2005d).
Note: Approximately $100 million of the total spent on lymphoma is allocated for non-Hodgkin lymphoma.

The choice of funding novel therapies, epidemiological studies, and clinical trials is necessarily more subjective than treatment *per se* as it is very much dependent on the pool of available investigators and their scientific interest. Innovation in research is often a matter of the success promised beforehand and in this regard certain research is more attractively pursued.

In 2005, more than twice as much money was allocated for breast cancer research as was allocated for lung and colorectal cancers even though the latter two claim five times as many lives. Pancreatic cancer is several times more deadly than melanoma and yet it attracts half as much funding, perhaps because it is so virulent. For some cancers, data on treatment costs are unavailable. Among these, only $11.7 million was devoted to stomach cancer research compared to $134.3 million for research on cancers of the brain and nervous system. The cancer business has no less bias than any other business:

> We think radiation therapy is the best, most cost-effective way to fight cancer, and we'd like to see that recognized. We're doing all the R&D work, but it's going to require a change of thinking in the medical community. (Varian Medical Systems 2004b)

Big corporations know all too well that there is no "best" way to treat cancer, because cancer is not a single disease. At the very least, the patient can only join the clinician in making an educated guess as to the ideal treatment under a very specific set of circumstances that will give the best quality of life.

Cancerous Tissues

Blood is a complex tissue serving as the body's transportation system. It is a highly nutritious protein-based solution that is 83% water by weight. Blood itself does not truly develop cancer and instead the disease develops where blood cells originate. Leukemia is cancer of the bone marrow—the spongy interior of most bones where red blood cells (cells that supply oxygen), white blood cells (cells that fight infection), and platelets (DNA-less cells that are needed for clotting) are formed and which upon maturing enter the circulatory system (also called the cardiovascular system) where they are suspended to function as the living part of the blood.

The lymphatic system is the body's immune system, a network of cells and organs that fight infectious diseases including cancer. Concentrated in the underarm, groin, neck, chest and abdomen, the lymphatic system includes the spleen, the thymus gland, tonsils, bone marrow, and lymph glands. Cancers of the lymphatic system refer to leukemia, lymphoma, myeloma, and sarcoma.

Table 6.1 compares the incidence of cancers whose primary site is not an organ but instead a type of tissue that may functionally be an organ, such as the skin, or part of a number of different organs. Basal cell and squamous cell

Table 6.1

New cases of tissue cancers diagnosed annually
per 100,000 population

Cancer	U.S.	Canada	Japan	U.K.
Basal cell and squamous cell	>335	210	-	111
Hodgkin lymphoma	2.6	2.6	-	2.4
Leukemia	11.8	12.4	5.1	9.7
Melanoma (skin)	20.9	13.6	(5.7)	11.9
Multiple myeloma	5.6	5.7	(2.9)	4.8
Non-Hodgkin lymphoma	19.8	19.9	-	12.9

Source: Jemal et al. (2006); Canadian Cancer Society (2006); National Cancer Center (2005); Cancer Research UK (2002); U.S. Central Intelligence Agency (2006).
Note: Rates are age-adjusted and (crude).

carcinomas are cancers of the skin caused by long-term exposure to the sun. They are for the most part easily treatable and not included as part of the world's cancer problem. The most common lymphatic cancers are leukemia (or leukaemia in Commonwealth English) and non-Hodgkin lymphoma, each accounting for 300,000 new victims annually worldwide (Mackay et al. 2006). Leukemia is also the most common childhood cancer in the world, and for reasons unknown, more prevalent in Caucasian peoples:

> Every hour of every day one person in the UK is diagnosed with lymphatic cancer. Around 45,000 people in the UK are living with the disease and incidence is rising. (Leukaemia Research 2005)

Melanomas are mostly cancers of the skin and far more of a health problem for light-skinned Caucasians than the darker-skinned Japanese killing 175,000 people annually worldwide (World Health Organization 2003). The development of melanoma is correlated with intense intermittent exposure to UV radiation over time, as occurs with severe sunburn, and not just from being in the sun. In fact, certain cancers, such as cancer of the breast, colon, and prostate gland, actually benefit from a daily exposure to sunlight (Kricker and Armstrong 2006). Melanoma occurs more frequently on the lighter colored palms and soles of dark-skinned people, whereas in whites, it is most commonly found on exposed parts—face, head, neck, and arm. Its origin is not well understood in that human skin is nearly a perfect absorber of radiation (less than 3% is reflected away and transmitted through it) showing no difference in race or complexion.

In the four countries followed here, leukemia and non-Hodgkin lymphoma claim the most lives (table 6.2). The World Health Organization (2005a) states that lymphomas and multiple myeloma account for 355,000 deaths per year worldwide; leukemia kills an additional 275,000 people of

Table 6.2

Yearly deaths from tissue cancers per 100,000 population

Cancer	U.S.	Canada	Japan	U.K.
Hodgkin lymphoma	0.5	0.3	(0.1)	0.4
Leukemia	7.5	6.6	3.8	5.2
Melanoma (skin)	2.7	2.7	(0.4)	2.4
Multiple myeloma	3.8	3.9	(2.8)	3.0
Non-Hodgkin lymphoma	6.3	9.1	(0.1)	5.5

Source: Jemal et al. (2006); Canadian Cancer Society (2006); National Cancer Center (2005); Cancer Research UK (2002); U.S. Central Intelligence Agency (2006).
Note: Rates are age-adjusted and (crude).

which 15,000 are 4 years and younger. Remarkably, melanoma skin cancer is more deadly in Japan than either lymphoma.

Cancers of the Skin

The skin is the body's largest organ and consists of several layers mainly classified as the epidermis or outer layer and the dermis or inner layer. The dermis is connective tissue and contains the blood and lymph vessels and is always protected by the harder epidermis that is epithelial tissue (layers of cells that cover the inside or outside surfaces).

Skin cancer begins in the epidermis and is either squamous cells, in the outer layer, basal cells, found just below the squamous, or melanocytes, which are the pigment (melanin) producing cells found in the inner layer, or located at the junction between the epidermis and the dermis. Melanoma is the deadliest skin cancer, a malignant tumor of the melanocytes that can also occur in the vagina and the iris (colored part) of the eye. The University of California, San Francisco warns that ionizing radiation may increase the risk of developing melanoma (Fink and Bates 2005). A single exposure to radiotherapy is reported to cause melanoma up to 45 years post-irradiation according to Shore (2001) of the New York University School of Medicine.

Localized melanomas are considered highly curable with surgery. Kirkwood and coworkers (1996) of the University of Pittsburgh claim that if the melanoma has spread to the lymph nodes implementing surgery with adjunctive interferon (proteins that boost the immune system) improves overall survival rates while chemotherapy does not. Chemotherapy is the treatment of choice for distantly metastasized stages of melanoma although overall survival is poor (Avril et al. 2004; Whitehead et al. 2004).

Basal cell and squamous cell carcinomas are usually found in middle-aged and older Caucasians and are associated with living in low latitude and exposure to UV, X-ray, and gamma radiation, and chemical carcinogens (Almahroos and Kurban 2004). These cancers are unlikely to spread through out the body and non-metastatic tumors are universally removed through excision, cryosurgery (sometimes called cryoablation), or laser surgery. On occasion radiotherapy is used for treatment when there is a concern for more favorable cosmetic results.

Merkel cell cancer is a rare skin cancer that is most commonly found in Caucasian men age 70 years and older. It too appears mostly in sun exposed areas like the head and neck and to a lesser extent the arms and legs (National Cancer Institute 2003a). Radical surgery seems to be about the only method of treating Merkel cell carcinoma. Pectasides, Pectasides, and Economopoulos (2006) reported poor prognosis due to the fact that nearly 30% of patients have regional lymph node metastasis at time of diagnosis ultimately developing distant metastasis within 2 years. A retrospective study of 68 male and 17 female Merkel cell cancer patients showed that while adjuvant radiotherapy had no effect on survival, it did in fact reduce recurrence. This study also demonstrated that females survived an average of 7.9 years compared to 6.4 years for males, the difference seemingly related to females being treated at a lower stage of the disease (Eng et al. 2004).

Ewing Sarcoma

Ewing sarcoma is typically manifested as a genetic malfunction according to the Paulussen, Frohlich, and Jurgens (2001) in Germany and Khoury (2005) of the Saint

Jude Children's Research Hospital in the United States. It is the second most common childhood cancer of the bone having an annual incidence of three per 1 million Caucasians and if the cancer is localized, surgery, chemotherapy, and radiotherapy are implemented but most Ewing sarcoma patients eventually succumb to distant metastasis (Paulussen, Frohlich, and Jurgens 2001).

The Saint Jude Children's Research Hospital adds that an intense chemotherapy regiment can provide 70% to 80% survival if the disease is localized with survival often reduced as a result of treatment-related complications leading to malignancies of the blood. Hematopoietic stem cell transplantation (bone-marrow replacement) is implemented for advanced stage patients in an effort to minimize metastasis but any relapse will ultimately be fatal (Rodriquez-Galindo 2004).

Complications associated with a combined treatment modality observed in 41 patients by the Mayo Clinic in Rochester, Minnesota over a 20-year period include "metastases, tumor recurrence, secondary malignancies, pathologic fractures, and radiation-associated and chemotherapy-associated morbidities" (Fuchs et al. 2003).

Hodgkin's Disease

Hodgkin's disease also called Hodgkin lymphoma spreads through the lymph nodes primarily located in the chest, the underarms, the groin, and in the abdomen. This cancer is diagnosed by its histology whereby cells appear larger than normal and contain pale nuclei.

According to the Mayo Clinic, Hodgkin lymphoma affects 7350 persons annually in the United States with the highest incidence among young adults and the elderly (Ansell and Armitage 2006). Hodgkin's disease is often associated with exposure to the Epstein-Barr virus—the primary cause of infectious mononucleosis, the so-called "kissing disease," and with HIV infections (Serraino et al. 2005). The Albert Einstein College of Medicine adds that HIV-associated Hodgkin's disease patients experience poor prognosis due to frequent lymph node involvement (Parekh, Ratech and Sparano 2003).

Several groups claim that 80% of all people stricken with this disease are cured with early stages (cancer limited to one lymph node region or two or more lymph node regions on the same side of the diaphragm) treated with chemotherapy or less commonly chemoradiotherapy (Connors 2005; Ng et al. 2004). In Europe, for example, chemotherapy regiments are considered the "gold standard"—the best available, widely accepted treatment— for early to intermediate stages delivering an 80% to 90% cure rate (le Maignan et al. 2004; Diehl et al. 2003). In Canada, radiotherapy treatments have reportedly declined concurrently with increased overall survival rates (Hodgson et al. 2003). Gustavsson, Osterman, and Cavallin-Stahl (2003) in Sweden and Connors (2005) in Canada treated advanced stages (cancer involves lymph nodes on both sides of the diaphragm or other organs besides the lymph system) Hodgkin's disease primarily with chemotherapy alone as neither group observed any evidence of any survival benefit with radiotherapy.

At all stages of the disease, there seems to be a greater risk of developing secondary malignancies, cardiac disease, and female breast cancer that is correlated with an increase in radiation exposure and the time lapsed after radiotherapy (Ng et al. 2002; Chronowski et al. 2003; Heidenreich et al. 2003; Horwich and Swerdlow 2004).

Kaposi's Sarcoma

Kaposi's sarcoma is a malignant tumor in the skin and mucus (viscous lubricating fluid) membranes of the mouth, nose, and anus. The human herpes virus-8 (HHV8) is detected in all forms of Kaposi's sarcoma according to a collaborative Canadian-American publication by Cheung, Pantanowitz, and Dezube (2005).

Prior to the early 1980's Kaposi's sarcoma was a rare disease found in elderly men of Mediterranean and Jewish ancestry ("classic"), young black African males ("African"), and patients undergoing immunosuppressive therapy related to kidney transplants ("transplant-related"). Recently a new form of Kaposi's sarcoma labeled as "epidemic" has increased in frequency as it is the most common malignancy associated with acquired immune deficiency syndrome (AIDS). However, homosexuals with and without AIDS have higher incidences of Kaposi's sarcoma indicating a non-AIDS related component to its origin (Gambus et al. 2001).

Classic Kaposi's sarcoma usually develops 10 to 15 years after the appearance of a benign tumor whereas African Kaposi's sarcoma is highly aggressive and 100% fatal within 3 years of its development. Due to the rarity of classic and African Kaposi's sarcoma it is difficult to find representative clinical trials that suggest a treatment of choice. However, radiotherapy is useful in treating both classic and African Kaposi sarcomas and for palliative purposes (Stein et al. 1993; Tombolini et al. 1999). When the classic disease has advanced, systemic (affecting the whole body) chemotherapy has achieved 33 months of additional life (Zidan et al. 2001).

According to a study in Spain, transplant-related Kaposi's sarcoma is typically associated with the immunosuppression procedure or by an Epstein-Barr viral infection that develops from the transplanted kidney itself. Post-operative patients are instructed to avoid sunlight and exposure to HBV and HCV to minimize the risk of Kaposi's sarcoma (Andres 2005).

Epidemic Kaposi's sarcoma affects approximately 20% of all homosexuals with AIDS and has declined in incidence with improvements in treatment. This malignancy steadily progresses from small local tumors to widespread dissemination and ultimately death. Epidemic Kaposi's sarcoma is associated with rapid disease progression and can kill the patient in less than 6 months (Cheung, Pantanowitz, and Dezube 2005).

A majority of recent studies focus on treatment for the two often incurable, rapidly spreading forms of Kaposi's sarcoma, epidemic and transplant-related. Life-threatening stages are treated with a "kitchen sink" approach—a combination of chemotherapy, radiotherapy, and immunotherapy (Dezube 2000 from Harvard and also Cattelan, Trevenzoli and Aversa 2002 from Padua, Italy) even when the soul purpose is palliation. Indeed, palliative radiotherapy is helpful for terminally ill AIDS patients who suffer from Kaposi's sarcoma as well as malignant lymphoma (Haas et al. 2003; Cheung, Pantanowitz, and Dezube 2005).

Promising results have been obtained with Highly Active Antiretroviral Therapy (HAART), a multichemical onslaught that suppresses virus replication until it is undetectable in the blood. HAART does not, however, improve patient survival (Nasti et al. 2003; Cheung, Pantanowitz and Dezube 2005).

Leukemia

Skeletal tissue, perhaps because there is no shortage of bone, is the second most likely site for cancer metastases. Males and females enter the world with approximately 270 bones that undergo a fusion process and reduce in number to 206 bones in adults. In bone, cancer may occur in the living cells that are imbedded in the rock-hard outer matrix as well as in the marrow-rich inner cavity.

Leukemia is cancer of the red bone marrow—the source of all blood found in the interior of most bones. All blood cells arise from primitive cells called stem cells. Table 6.3 gives the estimated breakdown of the four major leukemias: acute myeloid leukemia (AML), chronic lymphoblastic leukemia (CLL), chronic myelogenous or myeloid leukemia (CML), and acute lymphocytic leukemia (ALL). Often thought of as a childhood disease, leukemia is ten times more prevalent in adults. Table 6.3 shows also that all forms of leukemia are more common in males.

Table 6.3

Leukemia cases diagnosed annually in the United States

Leukemia	Male	Female
AML	6,350	5,580
CLL	6,280	3,740
CML	2,550	1,950
ALL	2,150	1,780

Source: Jemal et al. (2006).
Note: Statistics are age-adjusted.

Acute leukemias progress rapidly and characteristically target children whereas the chronic forms often take years to develop and are more common in older people. Leukemia has been linked to X-rays as early as 1911 and, with the exception of the CLL type, to atomic bomb radiation since 1945.

The most common form of adult leukemia is the stem cell disorder AML in which non-functional white blood cells called myeloblasts displace healthy blood cells and disrupt the process of fighting infection. According to Stone of the Dana-Farber Institute, in a published paper by Stone, O'Donnell, and Sekeres (2004), most people with AML will die of their disease. In California, O'Donnell of the City of Hope National Medical Center in the Stone, O'Donnell and Sekeres (2004) publication reports a median age of 68 years and 15% survival for those over the age of 60 years compared to 30% survival for younger adults. Stone in the same paper claims a greater 75% cure rate is achieved with AML patients in the 18 to 60 year age group through induction chemotherapy whereby all blood cell producing agents are removed from the marrow and repopulated with normal bone marrow cells. Bone marrow transplants may be implemented with augmented RIT in AML patients according to the Memorial Sloan-Kettering Cancer Center (Mulford and Jurcic 2004).

CLL is the second most common adult leukemia, a condition in which too many lymphocytes (another type of white blood cells) are produced. According to the University of Colorado Cancer Center, most people are older than 50 when diagnosed and all will ultimately succumb to other medical problems—not CLL. If the disease is advanced, survival is limited to less than 2 years. Although this disease progresses slowly and is not considered curable, treatment includes "watchful waiting" when few symptoms are exhibited, chemotherapy, localized radiotherapy, and stem cell transplants (Abbott 2006). Watchful waiting is a treatment option that literally means monitoring symptoms closely and postponing aggressive therapy unless symptoms of the disease progress.

Hairy cell leukemia—so-named due to the microscopic appearance of the malignant cells—is a rare form of CLL that based on work in Canada is considered easy to control with chemotherapy and without need for radiotherapy (Johnston et al. 2000).

CML is characterized by an increased production of myeloid cells, a type of stem cell. CML progresses slowly, rarely occurs in children, and is sometimes associated with prior exposure to ionizing radiation reports D'Antonio, a registered nurse and information specialist with The Leukemia & Lymphoma Society. The typical CML patient is 67-years old and diagnosed with a non-hereditary mutated gene (the fundamental unit of heredity composed of DNA). Median survival is a dismal 5 years. Chemotherapy with a remarkable drug called imatinib is the treatment of choice (D'Antonio 2005). Imatinib is an enzyme inhibitor that reduces the rate of cellular division. Some patients, however, eventually develop resistance to it, cautions the Texas M. D. Anderson Cancer Center (Cortes and Kantarjian 2005). Stem cell transplantation is recommended as an alternative by Lee and her coworkers (1998) at the Dana-Farber Cancer Institute in spite of a 15% to 30% probability of treatment related mortality.

ALL is related to having too many lymphocytes and has a causative relationship with the human T-lymphotropic virus type I (HTLV-I) (Proietti et al. 2005). This leukemia responds well to chemotherapy curing the majority of children and some adults although a fraction will suffer relapse or have a disease that resists therapy altogether (Blair et al. 2005). Similarly, the Saint Jude Children's Research Hospital in Tennessee reports 80% cure rates for ALL with a significant portion of the patients experiencing incurable relapse (Cheok, Lugthart, and Evans 2006).

Due to the fact that ALL is often hidden in the brain, the cranial nerves, and the spinal cord, cranial radiotherapy may be used. However, the Saint Jude Children's Hospital warns that exposing the patient's skull to radiation is not recommended for children due to the inherent 80% cure rate with chemotherapy alone (Pui et al. 2004). Others also note an increase in morbidity and growth stunting associated with treating this cancer with radiation (Darzy and Shalet 2003; Nathan et al. 2004).

Multiple Myeloma

Multiple myeloma is an incurable disease in which malignant white blood cells invade the bone marrow. As the bone marrow is attacked the outer layer of the bone is destroyed releasing an over-abundance of calcium into the bloodstream (hypercalcemia), causing severe bone pain and fractures that lead to kidney failure. The malignant cells also inhibit the growth of healthy white and red blood cells that can lead to anemia (too few red blood cells). It is a relatively rare and lethal cancer. In the United States, 9250 in men and 7320 in women will be diagnosed with this disease during 2006 and 5680 men and 5630 women are expected to die (Jemal et al. 2006).

Presently there is no known curative treatment for multiple myeloma and as such most attempts only prolong survival and reduce the symptoms according to the H. Lee Moffitt Cancer Center and Research Institute in Tampa, Florida (Kumar 2003). A number of groups in Europe report that high-dose chemotherapy and stem cell transplants are frequently employed to enhance survival (Sonneveld and Segeren 2003; Child 2003).

Localized radiation is only used palliatively. Experimental studies published in 2003 by Giralt and coworkers of the Texas M. D. Anderson Cancer Center and Breitz and coworkers of the NeoRx Corporation, a NASDAQ traded cancer therapeutics development company headquartered in Seattle, Washington demonstrated the use of short-lived (26.8-hours) holmium-166 to deliver high doses of 80 keV gamma and 666 keV beta radiation directly to the bone marrow via an organic phosphorus compound. Both groups noted this procedure is not without the risk of renal and bladder toxicity.

Myelodysplastic Syndromes

Myelodysplastic syndromes (MDS) are diseases of the bone marrow stem cells:

> Eighty percent of patients found to have MDS are older than 60 years and therefore not eligible for the only potentially curative therapy, bone marrow transplantation.... More than half of patients with MDS die within 2 to 4 years of infections, bleeding complications, or progression to acute [myeloid] leukemia. (Kurzrock 2002)

The Mayo Clinic has identified two types of MDS: *de novo* MDS occurring without any known cause and affecting mainly the elderly; and secondary MDS resulting from prior exposure to chemotherapy or radiotherapy (Steensma and Bennett 2006). Aul, Bowen, and Yoshida (1998) in Germany point out that while no one knows what causes MDS, risk factors include exposure to radiation and benzene, an ever-present petroleum product listed as a "known human carcinogen" and a cause of MDS, ALL, CLL, and Hodgkin lymphoma (Environmental Protection Agency 2003). It is also listed as a "potential occupational carcinogen" (Centers for Disease Control and Prevention (CDC) 2004b). Benzene is not going away anytime soon— the CDC (2006a) ranks benzene "in the top 20 chemicals for production volume" in the United States.

If a person with MDS is less than 50 years of age, stem cell transplants may be curative but not without the risk of 58% transplanted-related mortality according to Arnold and coworkers (1998) in Germany and Hofmann and coworkers (2004) of the UCLA School of Medicine in the United States. For the more typically older MDS patient and others who are not considered curable, treatment options include blood transfusions, immunosuppression therapy, and so-called investigational drug therapies (drugs only approved by the U.S. government for clinical trials and not general use) (Kurzrock (2002) of the M. D. Anderson Cancer Center; Steensma and Bennett (2006) of the Mayo Clinic).

Neuroblastoma

Neuroblastoma is a tumor that originates in nerve tissues of the neck, chest, abdomen, and most commonly around the paraspinal sites—the adrenal glands that are part of the kidneys. It is one of the most common solid tumors in children where in the United States approximately two thirds of those stricken are under 5 years of age. Worse yet, by the time symptoms become recognizable typically the tumors have already metastasized to lymph nodes, the liver, the lungs, and bone marrow reducing 5-year survival rates to as low as 45% according to a U.K. study (Cotterill et al. 2000). Survival decreases with the increasing age of the patient and tumor and the extent of involvement of the lymph nodes.

Rubie and coworkers (2001) in France and Garaventa et al. (2002) in Italy both claim that younger children with unresectable localized tumors treated with chemotherapy with or without surgery can have a greater than 90% 5-year overall survival rate. However, according to the Baylor College of Medicine in the United States there is a high rate of spontaneous regression with these tumors and due to the dangers of surgery, infants and small, localized tumors may be best treated with watchful waiting (Nuchtern 2006).

La Quaglia and coworkers (2004) of the Memorial Sloan-Kettering Cancer Center in the United States and von Schweinitz, Hero, and Berthold (2002) in Switzerland add that high-risk patients treated with surgery can expect overall survival rates of 50% even when distant metastasis has occurred especially when the patient is over 1 year of age.

The University of California, San Francisco reports that 539 high-risk neuroblastoma children treated with chemotherapy, surgery, and EBRT followed by more chemotherapy or bone marrow transplants combined with total body radiation were able to achieve 35% 5-year overall survival noting that radiotherapy improved local tumor recurrence and increased a need for intravenous feeding (Haas-Kogan et al. 2003).

The Memorial Sloan-Kettering Cancer Center in New York City reported after a more than 1-year follow-up investigation that IMRT was successful in treating 16 children to relieve pain symptoms without inducing myelopathy (functional disturbances of the spinal cord), although failing to show a reduction in tumor size (Bilsky et al. 2004).

Non-Hodgkin Lymphoma

Cancer originating in the lymphatic system is called lymphoma, and non-Hodgkin's disease, also called non-Hodgkin lymphoma (NHL), is the most common form of the disease. Like leukemia, NHL is more likely to strike elderly males and has been causally linked to immunosuppression, exposure to the human T-lymphotropic virus type I (HTLV-I), and Epstein-Barr virus (Muller et al. 2005).

There are more than two dozen clinically distinct types of NHL, a cancer that is more common than leukemia and ranks seventh in cancer incidence and mortality in the United States with new cases increasing at a rate of 3% to 4% per year in the 1970's and 1980's and beginning in the 1990's only 1% to 2% (Skarin and Dorfman (1997) of the Harvard Medical School; Muller et al. (2005) in Germany).

Adult NHL lymphomas that are slow growing and exhibiting few symptoms are said to be indolent. Treating these cancers with 35 Gy to 50 Gy radiation, Stanford University reported nearly 14-year median survival in 177 stage I (cancer found in one lymph node group or in a non-lymphatic organ) and stage II (cancer found on one side of the diaphragm or in an organ with lymph node involvement other than the primary lymph node site) NHL patients (Mac Manus and Hoppe 1996).

A retrospective analysis in the U.K. of 451 indolent and aggressive (lymphomas that grow and spread rapidly and which exhibit severe symptoms) stage I patients treated by radiotherapy resulted in 84% 10-year overall survival for those younger than 60 years of age at diagnosis (Vaughan Hudson et al. 1994).

Tondini and coworkers (1993) treated 183 aggressive stage I and II NHL patients with chemotherapy followed by adjunctive radiotherapy to achieve 83% overall 5-year survival, noting however, a higher relapse rate for radiotherapy than chemotherapy alone.

Watchful waiting is also recommended for intermediate (cancer found on both sides of the diaphragm) and advanced (cancer found in the lymph nodes and at least one organ) stage NHL patients by Multani, White, and Grillo-Lopez (2001) of Biogen Idec, Inc., a biotechnology corporation with 3000 plus employees in the United States and Ardeshna and coworkers (2003) in the U.K., who add that the median survival for indolent advanced stage cancer patients treated with chemotherapy is 5.9 years compared to 6.7 years for those denied immediate treatment. Treating aggressive intermediate and advanced stage NHL patients, the University Medical Center in Tucson, Arizona reported that chemotherapy plus radiotherapy improved 5-year overall survival from 82% compared to 72% for chemotherapy alone (Miller et al. 1998).

In France, Milpied's group (2004) and others have used high-dose chemotherapy followed by stem-cell support— the NHL patient uses healthy bone marrow to replace cells destroyed by the primary therapy—to treat people with NHL 15 to 60 years of age and concluded that the survival rate for patients at risk of death was significantly improved with this combination therapy. Most recently, the Mayo Clinic in

Minnesota reported that stem cell transplant was safely performed in patients over 60 years old to achieve a median survival of 25 months compared to a median survival of 56 months for younger people based on their study of 93 intermediate stage NHL patients treated from September 1995 to February 2003 (Buadi et al. 2006).

Waldenstrom's macroglobulinemia (WM) is another rare form of indolent NHL in which lymphocytes (white blood cells found in blood and lymph) multiply out of control and invade the bone marrow, lymph nodes, and spleen (the large reddish colored organ located on the left side of the body beneath the stomach filtering blood and providing antibodies).

In the United States there are

> 1,500 new cases annually ... [incidence] is higher in males and higher in whites than in African Americans. Incidence increases sharply with age. The median age at diagnosis is 63. (National Cancer Institute 2005c)

WM has no cure causing the body to produce an excess amount of the so-called IgM antibody that in turn causes the blood to thicken resulting in fatigue, a tendency to bleed easily, and a loss of circulation in the extremities. Treatment consists of first dealing with the blood thickening through a process by which the IgM antibody is removed from the blood. Then the underlying lymphoma is treated with either chemotherapy or interferon therapy, a form of immunotherapy. The UCLA Bone Marrow/Stem Cell Transplantation Program reported a promising 80% response rate in WM patients with low bone marrow involvement via RIT utilizing yttrium-90, a 2.28 MeV beta-emitting radioisotope with a 2.67-day half-life (Emmanouilides 2003).

Burkitt lymphoma is a rare form of pediatric NHL that is closely associated with the Epstein-Barr virus according to the Memorial Sloan Kettering Cancer Center (Gerecitano and Straus 2006). Burkitt lymphoma accounts for no more than 1% of all NHL and is mostly found in black African children who have a particular genetic defect although now it is also being sporadically diagnosed in blacks in the United States. This cancer has a tendency to spread rapidly and must be treated with intensive therapy administered over a short period according to the John Hopkins Hospital (Kasamon and Swinnen 2004). A 45-day multi-agent chemotherapy recipe was used in Italy to achieve 87% 5-year disease-free survival in children with stage III (extensive abdominal spread) and IV (bone marrow involvement) development (Spreafico et al. 2002).

NHL survivors face a 6% chance of developing a secondary tumor 3 to 20 years after first diagnosis. The most frequently observed secondary malignancies are Hodgkin's disease, AML, melanoma, and cancers of the brain, kidney, and bladder, whose occurrence appears related to the original NHL therapy (Travis et al. 1993).

Unfortunately, while prophylactic intercranial radiation at one time showed promise at mitigating tumor recurrence, it is no longer recommended due to the unacceptable morbidity associated with its administration (Gerecitano and Straus 2006).

Osteosarcoma

Osteosarcoma is the most common bone cancer in children and adolescents attacking the cells in the outer bone and what is often incorrectly thought of as non-living skeleton. Indeed, bone is very much alive—calcified connective tissue that is a surprising 22% water by weight. Osteosarcoma tumors form mostly at the ends of the long bones like the femur (thigh bone), the tibia (larger bone of the lower leg), and the humerus (upper arm bone) where they cause the joints to weaken and break. Height in adolescents is a risk factor (Longhi et al. 2005).

Most osteosarcoma patients have no known history to predisposition although it is positively linked to prior exposure to radiation, and in the rarer cases, to the same genetic abnormality that contributes to retinoblastoma (cancer of the retina) (Tabone et al. 1999). Since osteosarcoma readily spreads to other bones and the lung, survival is less than 30% even if the tumor is initially localized. Therefore, treatment almost always includes surgery followed by adjuvant chemotherapy.

A German study of 1702 children showed that osteosarcoma is very resistant to radiotherapy and thus the treatment of choice is multimodal chemotherapy, which in best case can give 10-year survival rates of up to 60%. Poor prognosis is associated with increased age, being male, tumor metastasis, and tumors that are incompletely removed by surgery (Bielack et al. 2002).

The Baylor College of Medicine in Houston, Texas retrospectively analyzed 30 studies of radiation-induced osteosarcoma evaluating the characteristics of 109 patients who were all less than 21 years of age at the time of diagnosis of the primary cancer. The researchers concluded that a dose of 15 Gy to 145 Gy induced osteosarcomas anytime 3 to 53 years post-radiotherapy. They also concluded that surgery plus adjuvant chemotherapy is the treatment of choice for patients with radiation-induced osteosarcomas providing a 68% 5-year overall survival rate (Koshy et al. 2005).

Soft Tissue Sarcoma

Cancers of the soft tissue are tumors that arise in the muscles, blood vessels, cartilage (connective tissue found at the joints and flexible parts of the nose and ears), tendons (connective tissue that connects muscle to bone), and fat, in fact, just about any tissue other than bone. Soft tissues vary greatly in both composition and density. Muscle and fat, for example, are approximately 76% and 30% water by weight respectively.

Devrup and Weiss (2006) of the Emory University in Georgia point out that soft tissue sarcomas present a special challenge to health care providers because staging does not lend itself to grading tumor development. The Texas M. D. Anderson Cancer Center adds that the cell structure of the soft tissue sarcoma is typically the most important prognostic indicator and even more so than the actual treatment (Zagars, Goswitz, and Pollack 2003).

Early stage soft tissue sarcomas are treated with surgery paying extreme attention to ascertaining that the malignant tumor is completely removed; otherwise local recurrence is inevitable. More advanced tumors risk local failure and distant metastasis requires combined adjuvant therapies to increase overall survival (Frustaci et al. 2001).

A Boston Massachusetts General Hospital study of 48 adults with 3-inch and larger tumors treated with preoperative chemotherapy combined with EBRT achieved 87% 5-year overall survival rates compared to 58% for those people left untreated. Nearly one third of those treated developed "wound complications" (DeLaney et al. 2003). Wound healing complications are also reported to occur with brachytherapy according to Ormsby and coworkers (1989) and more recently Spierer and coworkers (2003), all of whom are affiliated with the Memorial Sloan-Kettering Cancer Center.

Liposarcoma is a common soft tissue sarcoma found mostly in the lower extremities, a cancer that accounts for

fewer than 20% of soft tissue sarcomas ... the average patient ... is 50 years. In children, liposarcomas comprise fewer than 5% of soft tissue sarcomas. Fewer than 60 cases have been reported.... No racial predilection is apparent [and] two thirds of children with liposarcoma are boys.   (Konstantakos and Dudgeon 2002)

Surviving liposarcoma is highly dependent on identifying the tumor's histologic subtype (cellular structure) and less so on the treatment implemented.   Zagars, Goswitz, and Pollack (2003), for example, used surgery and adjuvant radiotherapy to achieve 90% local control and no metastasis in patients with well-differentiated cancer cells (cells that look noncancerous), whereas patients with pleomorphic cancer cells (cells without a distinctive shape) exhibited 37% local recurrence and all ultimately developed distant metastasis.

Rhabdomyosarcoma is a pediatric soft tissue cancer of the striated muscle (muscle attached to the skeleton) with tumors most commonly found in

the head and neck (28%), extremities (24%), and genitourinary (GU) tract (18%).... Approximately 250 cases [annually] ... 87% of patients are younger than 15 years, and 13% of patients are aged 15-21 years. (Cripe 2004)

The Duke University Medical Center reported treatment with surgery for localized tumors, surgery plus adjuvant radiotherapy for partially resected tumors, and chemotherapy for distant metastasis claiming that more that 70% of rhabdomysarcoma patients are cured. This is a most unusual claim in that there are very few cancers that are cured (eliminated with no likelihood of ever returning) (Breitfeld and Meyer 2005).

Angiosarcoma is a soft tissue cancer that originates in blood vessels and accounts for about 1% of all soft tissue sarcomas—some 60 cases per year in the United States. The Memorial Sloan-Kettering Cancer Center reported 31% 5-year survival rates for this cancer depending on how well the tumors were resected. Interestingly enough, tumor size does not seem to be a prognostic indicator (Fury et al. 2005).

Prior exposure to radiation is considered a risk factor for angiosarcoma. Of particular note, is the establishment by Stone and Holden (1997) of a causative link between the use of X-ray epiliation (hair-removal) therapy to treat scalp ringworm (*Tinea capitis*) in one child and its later development on the patient reaching adulthood. Brenn and Fletcher (2006) of the Brigham and Women's Hospital and Harvard Medical School, reported that the incidence of angiosarcoma is indeed rising and due in part to the increased use of radiotherapy to treat early stage breast cancer. Disturbingly, this is not a first time warning (e.g., Monroe, Feigenberg, and Mendenhall (2003) of the University of Florida College of Medicine in Gainesville, Florida. Here again, the perceived benefit of radiation as a cure-all for one cancer simply leads to an even more problematic cancer.

Three angiosarcoma patients were treated with some success using hyperfractionated (dividing the total dose of radiation into smaller doses that are administered more than once a day) EBRT followed by surgery. The result—"all 3 patients were alive without any recurrent disease 22, 38, and 39 months after treatment" (Feigenberg et al. 2002).

All Lousy Choices

Malignancies that originate in the four basic types of human tissue—epithelial, connective, muscle, and nervous—and are never confined to a single organ *per se* and instead spread throughout the body. These so called disseminated cancers have reasonable 5-year survival rates especially when diagnosed early (table 6.4).

Table 6.4

Five-year survival rates and preferred treatment
for cancers originating in a type of tissue

Cancer	Survival Rate (%)	Preferred Treatment
Ewing sarcoma	70	Chemotherapy
Hodgkin's lymphoma	85	Chemotherapy
Kaposi's sarcoma	57	HAART
Leukemia (ALL)	64	Chemotherapy
Leukemia (CLL)	74	Watchful waiting
Leukemia (AML)	21	Chemotherapy
Leukemia (CML)	44	Chemotherapy
Non-Hodgkin lymphoma	64	Radiotherapy (local + regional) Watchful Waiting or chemotherapy (late)
Melanoma (skin)	99 (local) 65 (regional) 15 (late)	Surgery (local + regional) Chemotherapy (late)
Multiple myeloma	33	Chemotherapy + Stem Cell Transplantation
Soft tissue sarcoma	66	Surgery (local + regional) Surgery + Chemotherapy or Radiotherapy (late)

Note: Survival Rates are 5-year relative survival rates (ratio of the proportion of cancer survivors to the proportion of expected survivors) taken from Ries et al. (2006); National Cancer Institute (2006e). Preferred Treatment is intended for informational purposes only, is not intended to constitute medical advice, and should not be relied upon in any such regard. Rates and treatment are not stage specific unless otherwise designated as: (local) cancer confined to the organ itself; (regional) cancer extending no further than surrounding tissue; and (late) cancer has metastasized to distant organs.

Localized treatments such as radiotherapy and surgery are not easily tailored to dealing with disseminated cancers and a systemic remedy like chemotherapy is usually required.

In spite of the difficulty of choosing a therapy to treat cancer, the state of Texas took it upon itself to add to the woes of the parents of a 13-year old girl diagnosed with Hodgkin's disease. A year ago the child's parents lost custody to Child Protective Services (CPS) for refusing to follow the advice of the M. D. Anderson Cancer Center: "the best course of treatment would be to follow the chemotherapy with radiation" (Wernecke 2005). When the parents argued that radiotherapy would do more harm than good, CPS asked a judge to "cut off all communication between the girl and her family" (Health Daily News Central 2005). The father simply noted, we "wanted to try other treatments for Katie before considering radiation as a last resort" (NewsTarget.com 2006).

Genital System Cancers

Cancer is more likely to strike the genital system of both sexes than anywhere else, although it is far more frequently found in men. In males, the prostate, testes, and penis are at risk. In females, cancer of the genitalia, also called gynaecological cancer, encompasses the cervix, uterus, ovaries, vulva, and vagina. Cancer of the cervix is the most frequently occurring genital cancer in the world, affecting 493,000 women annually (Mackay et al. 2006) and killing another 257,000 women each year (World Health Organization 2005a). It is not known why cancer of the genitalia is so prevalent.

The number of new cases of genital cancer diagnosed depends on who you are and where you live. Cervical cancer, which is four-times more prevalent in poor and developing countries, is infrequently found in countries such as the United States, Canada, and the U.K. where screening is routine (table 7.1). Almost all cervical cancers are caused by the sexually transmitted disease, human papillomavirus (HPV), even though the cancer itself is not

Table 7.1

New cases of cancer of the genital system diagnosed annually
per 100,000 population

Cancer	U.S.	Canada	Japan	U.K.
Cervix	3.3	4.1	-	8.4
Ovary	6.8	6.9	8.9	18.4
Penis	0.5	-	-	-
Prostate	78.7	62.5	21.7	91.3
Testis	2.8	2.5	-	6.5
Uterus	13.8	11.8	16.6	15.7
Vagina	0.8	-	-	-
Vulva	1.3	-	-	-

Source: Jemal et al. (2006); Canadian Cancer Society (2006);
National Cancer Center (2005); Cancer Research UK (2002);
U.S. Central Intelligence Agency (2006).
Note: Rates are all age-adjusted.

sexually transmitted or the least bit contagious. Viruses
that cause cancer are frequently referred to as oncogenic
and not carcinogenic. In the United States alone, more
than 20 million people are estimated to have genital HPV
and with millions more infected every year, an effective
vaccine against cervical cancer is unlikely. Moreover, with
as many as 200 distinct varieties of HPV known, and the
propensity of viruses to mutate and thereby survive, infect,
and replicate better, type-specific immunity is not
preventative. Nonetheless, the U.S. government has
recommended that all 11 to 12 year old girls be innoculated
(Centers for Disease Control and Prevention 2006c) with a
vaccine developed by Emory University that is said to be
100% effective for four distinctly different HPV infections,
two of which are oncogenic (Ault 2006).

Prostate cancer is a disease of the elderly, with an
incidence in Japan that is remarkably low compared to the
West. Studies have shown that Japanese men in Hawaii
have prostate cancer rates intermediate between those in

Japan and Caucasian Hawaiians. The difference suggests an environmental risk factor such as diet or physical inactivity. A high animal fat diet is frequently associated with high incidence whereas the frequency of ejaculation from sex, masturbation, and nocturnal emission appears to reduce the risk of developing prostate cancer (Leitzmann et al. 2004).

Prostate cancer is the deadliest genital cancer. Worldwide it kills 290,000 men per year, more than three-fourths of whom are 70 years and older (World Health Organization 2005a). Table 7.2 shows that in the United States, where prostate cancer is also the most commonly diagnosed cancer, mortality is relatively low, comparable to Japan, and in shocking contrast to the U.K. The disparity

Table 7.2

Yearly deaths from cancer of the genital system
per 100,000 population

Cancer	U.S.	Canada	Japan	U.K.
Cervix	1.2	1.2	(1.9)	2.8
Ovary	5.1	4.8	4.3	10.4
Penis	0.1	-	(0.1)	-
Prostate	9.2	12.7	8.5	26.6
Testis	0.1	0.1	(0.1)	0.3
Uterus	2.5	2.2	5.1	3.4
Vagina	0.3	-	(0.1)	-
Vulva	0.3	-	(0.1)	-

Source: Jemal et al. (2006); Canadian Cancer Society (2006); National Cancer Center (2005); Cancer Research UK (2002); U.S. Central Intelligence Agency (2006).
Note: Rates are age-adjusted and (crude).

between the U.S. and the U.K., a country with only 2% of its people black, is all the more remarkable since

> African American men have the highest rate of [prostate cancer] occurrence in the world and the lowest rate of survival. (Payne 2002).

Ovarian cancer kills 65% of all women afflicted in part due to its tendency to metastasize. The University of California, Irvine adds that 5-year survival rates are a dismal 20% to 30% worldwide (Tewari and DiSaia 2002). Ovarian cancer is especially common in Northern Europe with Scandinavia reporting the highest incidence in the world. This disease is associated with post-menopausal women who have never conceived and has been linked to the use of oral contraceptives. In the U.K. where 92% of the population is Caucasian and 4% is Asian (Indian and Pakistani), ovarian cancer is not only the most common gynecological cancer, it is also by far the deadliest.

Cervical Cancer

The cervix is the narrow opening extending from the uterus (womb), the place where the fetus develops, to the vagina, the opening of the uterus. Cervical cancer is a slow growing disease that does not typically give noticeable early signs. However, it is reliably detected with a Pap smear test (microscopic examination for abnormal cells). Invented by Georgios Papanicolaou, this screening method is so reliable that in the United States, a physician can be convicted of negligent homicide for failing to properly utilize this simple test to diagnose cervical cancer (The New York Times 1995). As with most cancers, early detection greatly improves prognosis. Stage I cervical cancers are confined to the cervix. Stage II and III cancers have spread beyond the uterus. In stage IV cancers, the disease has advanced beyond the pelvis (lower part of the abdomen).

At the very earliest stages, surgery is the treatment of choice. If surgery is not possible, brachytherapy alone is often recommended since EBRT does not consistently show a survival advantage (Chang et al. 2000 in Taiwan; Brewster et al. 2001 at the University of California, Irvine). In Italy, Frigerio and coworkers (1994) showed that adjunctive or adjuvant (not the primary treatment) radiotherapy after radical hysterectomy (surgical removal of the cervix, uterus and sometimes part of the vagina) actually increased patient morbidity with early stage cervical cancer candidates. However, 3 years later the same Italian university demonstrated that radiotherapy had no affect on patient morbidity (Landoni et al. 1997). In 1999, Tsai and coworkers in Taiwan reported 5-year overall survival rates of 76% in their study of early stage patients who received post-operative radiotherapy. Irradiating the pelvic area, as reported by Tsai's group, often causes small bowel injury wherein the lining of the small intestine becomes inflamed. This is commonly referred to as enteritis or enteropathy, a radiation sickness characterized by long-term diarrhea.

Resbeut and coworkers (2001) in France published a 7-year retrospective study of 192 women showing that brachytherapy prior to a hysterectomy gave a 91% 5-year disease free survival for stage I and II. A 20-year long U.S. retrospective study of 185 women treated with EBRT followed by brachytherapy demonstrated a 5-year disease free survival of 67%, 49%, and 17% in stage II, III, and IV respectively (Syed et al. 2002). Similarly, the Mallinckrodt Institute of Radiology in Saint Louis, Missouri demonstrated very similar success although roughly half of their patients suffered recurrence and metastasis (Grigsby et al. 2001).

In general, there are many side affects including vaginal and bladder morbidity that are associated with utilizing radiation for cervical cancer due the compactness of organs in the pelvic area (Resbeut et al. 2001; Grigsby et al. 2001; Yalman et al. 2002). A Japanese study of 177 women with stage I to III cervical cancers treated by EBRT combined with brachytherapy (radium-226, a gamma emitter with a 1603 year half-life) between 1986 and 1995 resulted in treatment failure due to distant metastases (16%) and tumor recurrence in the pelvis (11%) (Sasaoka et al. 2003). A larger 827 patient Japanese study conducted 2 years earlier indicated higher incidences of tumor recurrences in patients treated by radiotherapy (7.1%) compared to those who underwent surgery (1.2%) (Takehara et al. 2001).

The University of Kentucky Medical Center reported in 1991 actuarial 10-year survival rates of 87%, 61%, and 25% for stage I, II, and III cancers respectively using neutron brachytherapy (NBT) explaining in a publication 2 years later that because the NBT implants caused the tumors to regress so rapidly, the adjacent organs (bladder, rectum, colon, and bowel) suffered excess radiation exposure (Maruyama et al. 1991; 1993). More recently a group in the Czech Republic reported that californium-252 NBT gave 19% better overall 5-year survival rates than the more "conventional" gamma emitting brachytherapy (Tacev, Ptachova, and Strnad 2003).

Combining chemotherapy with radiotherapy is used to treat the local recurrence and distant metastasis that so often accompanies this disease. Benedetti-Panici and coworkers (2002) in Italy, for example, conducted a randomized trial of 441 stage I to III and found a 59% 5-year overall survival rate for patients treated with chemotherapy prior to radical surgery compared to 45% for patients assigned to EBRT followed by brachytherapy. The M. D. Anderson Cancer Center achieved a 67% 8-year overall survival rate with cisplatin enhanced pelvic radiotherapy compared to only 41% with extended field (irradiating the tumor and the surrounding area) radiotherapy alone (Eifel et al. 2004). Maduro and coworkers (2003) in the Netherlands add that radiotherapy causes toxicity to surrounding organs and tissue and leads to secondary malignancies developing for more than 20 years after treatment. Enhancing the radiation therapy with cisplatin markedly increased blood toxicity without affecting other side effects.

Ovarian Cancer

The ovary is the egg-producing organ. Located in the pelvis (between the hip bones) on either side of the uterus each ovary is an endocrine or ductless gland that secretes estrogen (a sex hormone responsible for secondary sex characteristics) and progesterone (a steroid hormone involved in menstruation and pregnancy).

The most common cancer of the ovary is epithelial (organ covering tissue) ovarian carcinoma, which is the cause of one-fifth of all cancer deaths in women. The majority of women are over 65 years of age and 5% to 10% of them have a family member also with the disease. Partly due to the fact that the cancer shows very little symptoms at the time of diagnosis the surrounding lymph nodes are usually invaded and the woman's prognosis is poor.

A far less common ovarian cancer known as a Krukenburg tumor is a secondary cancer that is frequently a consequence of cancer in the stomach or the colon— literally a metastatic stomach or colon cancer that has traveled to the uterus.

For women with early stage I (growth limited to the ovaries) or stage II (some extension into the pelvis) disease, surgery is the best option ranging from the removal of the ovary to a total hysterectomy. If the tumor is found in both ovaries or has spread to the uterus or the fallopian tubes, which connect the two, surgery is not a sufficient cure. Additional treatment options include intraperitoneal (chemically administered directly through the abdomen) phosphorus-32 radiotherapy, high-dose whole abdominal radiation therapy (WART), and systemic (treatment via the bloodstream) chemotherapy. None of these methodologies, however, have demonstrated a survival advantage.

Clinical trials by Vergote and coworkers (1992) in Norway and Young's group (2003) in the United States comparing chemotherapy with the slow infusion of phosphorus-32, a pure beta-emitting radioisotope with a 14.3 day half-life, into the patient's abdomen concluded that although a 75% 5-year survival rate could be achieved in early stage patients with well-developed tumors, the phosphorus-32 radiotherapy was not recommended due to late bowel complications.

A recent Italian study of 477 women with ovarian cancer in five European countries has suggested that platinum-based chemotherapy used in conjunction with surgery can increase the 5-year survival rate for early stage patients from 70% without chemotherapy to 79% with chemotherapy (Colombo et al. 2003).

Once the cancer has reached stage III (tumor extends no further than the bowels) or stage IV (disease shows distant metastasis), a total hysterectomy along with the ovary becomes the minimum therapy required. More typically, at least according to the Fox Chase Cancer Center in Philadelphia, chemotherapy will be used either before or after surgery to reduce the tumor size. However, due to the high likelihood of tumor recurrence, the overall survival in advance-stage ovarian cancer patients remains at less than 5 years (Varia et al. 2003; Ozols et al. 2003).

A retrospective U.S. study of WART of 71 women with ovarian cancer yielded 5-year survival rates of 93%, 48%, and 29% in stage I, II, and III, respectively (Firat, Murray, and Erickson 2003). These impressive results are deemed comparable to the most successful systemic chemotherapy and yet, a systematic overview of 1282 women in Sweden concluded that there is no scientific evidence showing that radiotherapy used in conjunction with surgery offers a benefit for early stage ovarian cancer (Einhorn et al. 2003).

According to the Texas M. D. Anderson Cancer Center, tumors of the stromal cell (cells that produce hormones) and germ cell (cells that produce eggs) account for less than 10% of all ovarian cancers. Stromal tumors occur most frequently in women aged 40 to 60 years while germ cell tumors are most common in teenagers. And in both cases, the "gold standard" of treatment is post-operative chemotherapy which can achieve a truly remarkable 95% overall disease-free survival rate (Gershenson 1993).

Penile Cancer

The penis, like most all other organs, comes in different shapes and sizes. Cancer of the penis is extremely rare in the developed world and in Western countries in particular. Whenever it occurs the dominant risk factor is associated with males who are not circumcised (surgical removal of the foreskin from the penis) as infants and in men who exercise poor genital hygiene. It is noteworthy that more than 80% of the world does not practice circumcision and in the United States less than 60% of the newborn males are circumcised today compared to 90% in 1979.

The 5-year overall survival rates for penile cancer patients treated with surgery and adjuvant radiotherapy ranges from 22% to 70%, according to a Taiwanese study depending mostly on whether distant metastasis has occurred in the lymph nodes of the groin (Chen et al. 2004). In those cases, the best control of distant metastasis seems to be associated with the surgical removal of the lymph nodes in the groin as chemotherapy shows no efficacy (Pow-Sang et al. 2002).

For local tumor control, treatment options include amputation of the penis (Singh and Khaitan 2003), interstitial brachytherapy (Crook et al. 2002; Singh and Khaitan 2003), and laser ablation (vaporizing the tumor) (Singh and Khaitan 2003; Windhal and Andersson 2003), of which the latter most penile cancer treatment appears to afford the best cosmetic results, if indeed there is such a thing.

A 1962 to 1994 Swiss study of 41 men with penile cancer indicated that better local tumor control was obtained with surgery versus radiotherapy, although there was no difference observed in overall survival rates (Zouhair et al. 2001). There appears to be no argument that irradiating the penis can cause tissue death, infection, testicular damage, and metastasis.

Prostate Cancer

The endocrine system refers to all of the body's ductless glands—organs that secrete hormones directly into the bloodstream. The prostate gland is one of the body's endocrine glands. It is a walnut-sized male only organ that sits just below the urinary bladder. It produces the seminal fluid that accompanies sperm during orgasm or ejaculation. Innocuous for most of its life the prostate gland tends to enlarge in old age and obstruct the urethra (the genital duct from which urine and semen passes) sometimes necessitating its removal.

The overall survival rate of prostate cancer patients is like most cancers directly related to the size and extent of the cancerous tumor. If the tumor is confined to the prostate (stage I and II also termed stage A or B in the Whitmore-Jewitt staging system), survival is greater than 5 years. Stage III cancer (equivalent to stage C in the

Whitmore-Jewitt system) that has spread outside the prostate and may invade the seminal vesicles by which semen is produced is currently not considered curable. If the cancer has spread to the lymph nodes or distant organs such as the liver and the lungs (stage IV or D in the Whitmore-Jewitt system) survival is reduced to just 1 to 3 years. Thus there is great impetus to diagnose prostate cancer early and implement curative treatment expeditiously.

A test for prostate specific antigen (PSA) is often used to screen for this disease. However, a high PSA level in the blood does not necessarily indicate cancer as it is also associated with natural aging, prostatis (inflammation), and benign prostatic hyperplasia (a noncancerous enlargement of the gland). A biopsy is always required to prove cancer:

> If the purpose of the PSA test is to make a decision for radical prostatectomy ... for radiotherapy ... for chemotherapy, it is a poor test. But, if the purpose ... is to assess prostate health, the PSA test is the most practical, cheapest, and useful test. If the purpose ... is to monitor the efficacy of a cancer control program, it is more valuable than most types of scans for the prostate gland. (Ali 2005)

Watchful waiting is a highly recommended treatment option for prostate cancer in its earliest stages. A 1977 to 1984 Swedish study of 642 prostate cancer patients concluded that those men with localized tumors (stage I and II) can have a favorable outlook simply by following a watchful waiting approach and thereby avoiding the potential deaths brought about by "radical" initial treatment (Johansson et al. 1997):

> By dramatically strengthening the body's immune system through diet, nutritional supplements, and exercise, the body can rid itself of the cancer, just as it

does in other degenerative diseases. Consequently, I wouldn't have chemotherapy and radiation because I'm not interested in therapies that cripple the immune system, and, in my opinion, virtually ensure failure for the majority of cancer patients. (Whitaker 2003)

If it is determined that watchful waiting is no longer an option, men with prostate cancer who are in good health and those over 70 years old typically are offered the option of surgery which first may entail a radical prostatectomy (surgical removal of the prostate gland, surrounding tissue, and nearby lymph nodes). A 15-year Johns Hopkins Hospital study of 2404 men showed that for clinically localized prostate cancer, surgery achieved overall actuarial (statistical) 5-year and 10-year recurrence-free survival rates of 84% and 74%, respectively (Han et al. (2001).

Hull and coworkers (2002) published a 15-year study that showed that 75% of 1000 early stage prostate cancer patients who had undergone surgery as a curative treatment were likely to remain free of any cancer for at least a decade. And according to the Yale Medical School, very little post-operative complications have been catalogued for resected (surgically removed) cancer patients. In fact, less than 10% of the men so treated were found to suffer urinary incontinence (inability to prevent urine loss) and 48% to 69% retained their sexual potency (Peschel and Colberg 2003).

EBRT is a treatment option offered at all stages of this disease while brachytherapy is implemented if the cancer has not spread outside the prostate. Clinical studies, however, do not support their efficacy. A British study of 999 patients who were treated with radiotherapy showed survival rates of 22% to 79% depending on how far advanced the prostate cancer had been diagnosed adding that if the cancer has not spread outside the prostate there is no benefit to using radiation in addition to surgery (Duncan et al. 1993). About 80% of the men diagnosed with prostate cancer in the United States have early stage disease and

> there are no randomized trials that compare the relative benefits of treating early stage patients with radiation therapy, radical prostatectomy, or watchful waiting.... It is not known ... if surgery is better than radiation, or if treatment is better than no treatment in some cases. (National Cancer Institute 2003b)

And in 2001, the British Council, a non-profit organization established in 1934, remarked that

> the survival rate for patients with well and moderately differentiated [prostate] tumors are identical whether they are managed by radiotherapy or by watchful waiting.

While no life-threatening complications appear to accompany pelvic radiotherapy treatments for prostate cancer, IMRT was explored at the University of Chicago as a means of escalating the dose while minimizing acute toxicity of the penile bulb (base of the penis) and the surrounding radiation sensitive tissues (Jani, Roeske, and Rash 2003). And while prostate cancer is today the single most common cancer treated with IMRT, the requisite tumor modeling has yet to fully exploit its potential. Considering then that a typical IMRT treatment lasts between 15 and 30 minutes, it is easy to understand the difficulties of confining the radiation to such a small target in a not so quiescent living patient as encountered at the Fox Chase Cancer Center in Philadelphia:

Prostate position may be influenced by differences in daily patient setup, rectal filling, bladder filling, and even respiration. (Pollack et al. 2003)

In spite of these inherent difficulties, the Memorial Sloan-Kettering Cancer Center in New York City reported that 772 clinically localized prostate cancer patients treated with 81 Gy to 86 Gy IMRT between April 1996 and January 2001 had reduced acute and late rectal and urinary toxicities relative to conformal EBRT (Zelefsky et al. 2002). The Sloan-Kettering study did not, however, make any comparison to non-irradiated cancer patients nor did it provide any overall survival rates.

Brachytherapy is another recommended radiation treatment for a wide range of prostate cancer conditions. A comprehensive study from the M. D. Anderson Cancer Center Orlando in Orlando, Florida evaluated 2991 localized prostate cancer patients treated with surgery, brachytherapy seeds, EBRT, or a combination of EBRT and brachytherapy, and concluded that no advantage was shown for any radiation treatment over surgery in terms of overall survival rates or subsequent biochemical tests such as PSA detection (Kupelian et al. 2004).

In men with advanced stage tumors where the cancer has spread beyond the prostate to nearby tissues and possibly the seminal glands (organs that help produce semen) surgery may not be an option. A remarkably low 7 Gy EBRT study of 372 inoperable stage III patients in the United States proved beneficial: 245 men were alive 5 years after treatment, 142 after 10 years, 64 after 15 years, and 24 after 20 years (del Regato, Trailins, and Pittman 1993).

In the highest risk prostate cancer patients, those exhibiting metastasis, combined radiotherapy and brachytherapy is often implemented. Even then, however, a 10-year study by the Seattle Prostate Institute in which 45

Gy EBRT was combined with palladium-103 and/or iodine-125 seeds resulted in higher post-treatment complications without demonstrating any therapeutic benefit to the patient compared to brachytherapy alone (Blasko et al. 2000). While not a welcome result, a 15-year U.S. study investigating the use of iridium-192 seed brachytherapy (30 Gy) in conjunction with EBRT (36 Gy) drew the same conclusion (Puthawala et al. 2001).

So while radiotherapy does not yet appear to improve the overall survival rates for men with prostate cancer, in particular those with localized tumors, the detrimental affects of radiation exposure must be considered:

> Radical surgery or radiotherapy can cause harm (commonly impotence and/or incontinence) and have not yet been shown to reduce prostate cancer mortality. (British Council 2001)

No difference across the Atlantic:

> Most cases of prostate cancer that are being discovered with present methods are not fatal. Moreover, aggressive treatment of prostate cancer confers substantial risk for illness and a small but finite risk for death.... No published controlled trials have proven that radical prostatectomy or radiotherapy reduces rates of death from clinically localized prostate cancer. (American College of Physicians 1997)

The very nature of brachytherapy requires that the tumor be localized and in close proximity to the radioactive source. Therefore it is not too surprising that the Yale Medical School published a review paper summarizing that "the best candidates for radical prostatectomy are also the best candidates for implant therapy," noting further that about 2% to 18% of all stage I and II prostate cancer patients undergoing brachytherapy develop complications that require simple outpatient treatment or require major surgical intervention and possibly long hospital stays. Post-brachytherapy complications include urinary incontinence, urinary retention (difficulty urinating), urethral strictures (abnormal narrowing of the urethra), urethritis (inflammation of the urethra characterized by painful urination), cystitis (inflammation of the bladder also associated with painful urination), prostatitis (inflammation of the prostate characterized by irregular urination), proctitis (inflammation of the rectum characterized by bloody stool and frequent need to defecate), rectal ulceration (wounds in the rectum) and rectal fistula (incomplete closure of such a wound) (Peschel and Colberg 2003).

One of the major side effects of using radiotherapy to treat prostate cancer is acute rectal toxicity, a condition characterized by bleeding and pain. A Texas M. D. Anderson Cancer Center study of 305 men diagnosed with early stage prostate cancer reported that higher doses of radiation correlated with rectal side effects and without giving any survival benefit (Pollack et al. 2002). In addition, the Harvard Medical School adds that bladder toxicity and hematuria (blood in the urine) often accompanies post-radiotherapy and is present as late as 20 years after exposure (Gardner et al. 2002). And finally, Sloan-Kettering's Zelefsky and coworkers (2002) among others have documented side effects from IMRT that include rectal toxicity, acute urinary symptoms, urinary retention, and urinary toxicity.

According to a massive 1994 to 1995 NCI compilation of several thousand men living in major U.S. metropolitan areas and diagnosed with localized prostate cancer and treated with EBRT:

> Sexual function is the most adversely affected following external radiation beam therapy, with problems

continuing to increase between 12 and 24 months post-radiation. Bowel function problems increased at six months but were partially resolved by 24 months. (National Cancer Institute 2003b)

More than 10 years ago, the University of Miami School of Medicine observed that 136 prostate cancer patients who underwent radical prostatectomy complained of worsened urinary incontinence and sexual function following surgery, whereas 60 men treated with EBRT complained of having problems with bowel functionality after treatment (Lim et al. 1995). Shortly thereafter, the Fox Chase Cancer Center in Philadelphia was quick to point out that chronic rectal bleeding of severity requiring blood transfusions and/or coagulations is another complication associated with conformal radiotherapy and that this complication worsened with escalating radiation dose (Hanlon et al. 1997). A more recent University of Southern California study of nearly 500 men with localized prostate cancer who underwent EBRT concluded that 43% of the men who claimed being sexually potent before radiation exposure became impotent 2 years after treatment (Hamilton et al. 2001).

A 20-year long (1973-1993) Columbia University, New York retrospective study of 51,584 prostate cancer patients treated with radiotherapy compared to 70,539 patients treated with surgery showed that 0.34% of those exposed to radiation risked developing a secondary tumor in the bladder, rectum, lung, and even in the treated area itself. Moreover, if the person survived for 10 or more years, the secondary tumor risk associated with radiotherapy increased by 34% (Brenner et al. 2000).

An option for prostate cancer patients who are too old or too ill is called transurethral resection of the prostate (TURP), a procedure in which prostate tissue is removed using a thin tube inserted through the urethra into the penis. TURP is primarily used for noncancerous prostates and thus only treats the symptoms of the disease by removing a part of the tumor.

Lastly, hormone therapy is sometimes used alone or in conjunction with surgery or radiation to shrink the tumor or slow its growth. Hormone therapy works by blocking the action of testosterone (steroid hormone associated with secondary sex characteristics) either by surgically removing the testicles or by introducing antiandrogens (drugs that interfere with male sex hormones) directly into the bloodstream. It is notable that antiandrogens do not prevent the production of testosterone and so they do not cause impotence whereas surgical castration is permanent and the patient is forever impotent.

Testicular Cancer

The testes are a pair of endocrine glands housed in the scrotum (an external sac) and are a primary cancer site. The testes form in the abdominal cavity and descend into the scrotum before birth. After adolescence the testis produces sperm and generates testosterone that is critical for prostate gland cancer to develop and grow.

Testicular cancer is most prevalent in affluent Caucasian males with late descending testicles and in men with familial testis cancer. In the United States,

> testicular cancer occurs most often in men between the ages of 20 and 39, and is the most common form of cancer in men between the ages of 15 and 34. It is most common in white men, especially those of Scandinavian descent. (National Cancer Institute 2005a)

Almost all forms of this cancer begin in the germ (reproductive) cells of the testicles where immature sperm first develop and consist of two main types of tumors—

seminomas and nonseminomas. Seminomas account for less than half of all testicular cancers and are most common in older adults while the more prevalent nonseminomas usually develop in younger males.

If a person develops a tumor in one testicle they are more than 25 times more likely to develop a second tumor in the other testicle (Colls et al. 1996). According to a 51-year Memorial Sloan-Kettering Cancer Center study of 3984 testicular cancer patients, the development of this secondary tumor was more likely in seminomas and typically occurred within 50 months of the discovery of the original seminoma (Holzbeierlein, Sogani, and Sheinfeld 2004).

For all those with testicular cancer, the treatment of choice is an orchiectomy (surgical removal of one or both testicles) and as a consequence of removal, the loss of a major source of male hormones—a difficult decision to say the least. Alternatively, early stage nonseminoma cancer patients are also successfully treated with adjuvant chemotherapy or lymph-node dissection. It is impossible to evaluate the "best" remedy as survival is nearly 100% irrespective of the initial treatment (Jones and Vasey 2003).

Since seminomas are well known to be radiation sensitive the "gold standard" for treating them is surgery followed by radiotherapy (Scholz and Holtl 2003). The M. D. Anderson Cancer Center claims that surgery plus EBRT provides 93% and 79% 10-year and 20-year survival rates respectively in stage I (cancer confined to the testicle) and II (disease includes blood and/or lymph involvement). In spite of these impressive results, serious consideration is given to the excessive risk of secondary cancers, cardiac disease, and damage to the genetic material associated with exposing the testes to radiation (Zagars et al. 2004).

Extragonadal germ cell tumors are not located in the testicles and are believed to develop from embryonic testicular cells that travel to another part of the body, typically the chest or the abdomen. Accounting for less than 5% of all germ cell tumors, the cancerous form is very rare and aggressive and is usually found in young males. Interestingly enough, extragonadal nonseminomas have a higher likelihood of developing a secondary testicular cancer later in the person's life than do extragonadal seminomas (Bokemeyer et al. 2003).

As with testicular seminomas, the extragonadal germ cell seminomas are particularly sensitive to radiotherapy and if the tumor is localized to the mediastinum (the chest part extending from the neck to the heart and not including the lungs), cure rates as high as 60% to 75% are achieved with radiotherapy. However, seminomas that are too large or have metastasized are generally treated with chemotherapy (Clamon 1983).

The nonseminoma extragonadal germ cell tumors are not very sensitive to radiation nor are they easily surgically removed. Men with nonseminomas are most likely treated with chemotherapy and have a poor prognosis due to tumor recurrence and metastasis. One German group published a retrospective study reporting 5-year survival rates for nonseminomas treated with chemotherapy that ranged from 17% to 69%, with the poorer prognosis being associated with tumors located in the center most part of the chest—the most likely location and often accompanied by metastasis to the liver, lung, or central nervous system (Hartmann et al. 2002).

Uterine Cancer

For all of us, life begins in the uterus, the pear shaped organ that connects the vagina to the ovaries. Tumors of the uterine corpus (upper part of the uterus) include an endometrial form and a rarer type called uterine sarcoma that accounts for no more than 5% of all uterine cancers.

Endometrial carcinoma involves the lining of the uterus and is often caused by the use of the steroid, estrogen as a replacement hormone, or the use of tamoxifen (an anticancer drug that blocks the effects of estrogen) as a chemotherapeutic agent for breast cancer (Carter and Pather 2006). Women with high-blood pressure, who are obese, or infertile, are also at the highest risk for the endometrial form. Like ovarian cancer, the risk of developing uterine cancer is reduced in women who use oral contraceptives particularly ones in which the estrogen and progesterone are in balance. White women are more typically diagnosed with lower grade tumors than black women and consequently experience better survival (Reddy et al. 1997).

According to the University of Virginia Health System, the 5-year survival rate for early stage I (cancer is in the uterus and not in the cervix) is 83% to 93%; for intermediate stage II (cancer has spread to the cervix) it is 73%; for late stage III (cancer is confined to the pelvis and not advanced to the bladder or rectum) it is 52%; and for metastatic stage IV it is 27% (Irvin, Rice, and Berkowitz 2002).

Early stage cancer of the endometrium (mucus membrane that lines the uterus) is commonly treated with a hysterectomy. Remarkably, even the complete removal of the uterus via a hysterectomy does not preclude its later development as the cancer may have already metastasized to other organs. The importance of removing the fallopian tubes and both ovaries cannot be over emphasized, as these organs are common metastatic sites (Carter and Pather 2006).

A randomized Dutch study of 715 patients with early stage endometrial carcinoma determined that adjuvant EBRT fails to give a "survival benefit" and that radiation exposure increases complications with the urinary and gastrointestinal (stomach and intestines) tracts persisting in half the patients for up to 5 years at least (Creutzberg et al. in 2001). Three years later this same research group showed that after nearly 7 years post-radiotherapy follow-up the risk of distant metastases was not eliminated (Creutzberg et al. 2004).

A British study of 228 stage I endometrial carcinoma patients post-operatively treated with EBRT, brachytherapy, both radiotherapies, or no radiotherapy at all, published in 2003 by Moss and coworkers showed 90% 5-year overall survival rates. Similarly, a same year University of Alabama Hospital at Birmingham study of 220 stage I patients concluded that radiotherapy had no effect on survival (Straughn et al. 2003). And Herwig and coworkers (2004) of the University of Innsbruck, Austria observed late cases of urinary incontinence in more than half of their stage I patients treated with either EBRT or brachytherapy.

It is universally experienced by research groups worldwide that endometrial carcinoma patients classified as intermediate risk stage II and III do not show a significant improvement in overall survival rates when post-operative EBRT or brachytherapy is implemented primarily because the distant metastasis problem is not addressed (Touboul et al. 2001 in France; Jereczek-Fossa 2001 in Poland; Keys et al. 2004 in the United States; Ayhan et al. 2004 in Turkey).

In California, the Stanford University School of Medicine claimed 3-year 89% overall survival rates in stage III or IV endometrial carcinoma patients treated post-operatively with WART, noting that failures were a result of the ever-present distant metastasis (Smith et al. 2000). Attempting to deal with this problem, Randall, Spirtos, and Dvoretsky (1995) at the Indiana University Medical Center, compared chemotherapy to WART in a post-operative study of 422 advanced stage patients and found chemotherapy had better overall survival, 7% less gastrointestinal tract toxicity, and 15% less damage to the heart.

The rare uterine sarcoma is described as tumors growing in the muscles or supporting tissues of the uterus. Women with uterine sarcoma have a median age of 60 years, a stage I 5-year survival rate of 50%, and are more commonly black (Reddy et al. 1997). One possible cause of this cancer is a one time exposure to radiation:

> The only documented etiologic [study of causes or origins] factor in 10% to 25 % of these malignancies is prior pelvic radiation, often administered for benign uterine bleeding 5 to 25 years earlier. (National Institute of Cancer 2006c)

It is not clear how effective post-operative adjuvant radiotherapy is in increasing the overall survival rates of women with uterine sarcoma. A Spanish study of stage I to stage IV uterine sarcoma patients showed that 5-year overall survival rates improved from 37% to 73% using 48 Gy total WART, with and without brachytherapy (Ferrer et al. 1999). A University of Vienna, Austria group combined 56 Gy EBRT with 21 Gy brachytherapy to treat 72 uterine sarcoma patients achieving 75% 5-year survival rates in stage I, 53% in stage II, 16% in stage III, and zero survival in stage IV (Knocke et al. 1998). Nonetheless,

> adjuvant radiation decreases local recurrence rates for uterine sarcomas, but has not been clearly shown to improve overall survival. (Hensley 2000)

The University of Pittsburgh, Pennsylvania agrees with Sloan-Kettering explaining that adjuvant radiotherapy certainly can reduce the local recurrence of uterine sarcoma tumors but is ineffective in destroying tumors that have spread outside the uterus and which will ultimately result in death (Gerszten et al. 1998).

Vaginal Cancer

The vagina is a muscular 3 to 6-inch long multipurpose tube that connects the uterus to the outside world. It is capable of stretching itself several times its size as during intercourse and childbirth. Cancer of the vagina is fortunately uncommon. However, women with an earlier hysterectomy or prior exposure to pelvic radiation have a higher risk of developing vaginal cancer. The majority of vaginal cancers are squamous cell carcinomas (tumors with cells that have a flat, scaly appearance and develop in the lining of the vagina). These often metastasize to the lungs and the liver and are related to the sexually transmitted human papillomavirus (HPV) which is now listed as a "known carcinogen" by the U.S. government:

> For the first time ever, viruses are listed in the report: hepatitis B virus, hepatitis C virus, and some human papillomaviruses that cause common sexually transmitted diseases. (National Institute of Environmental Health Sciences 2005a)

Approximately 15% of the remaining vaginal cancers are adenocarcinomas that generally occur in women 21 years and younger and which metastasize to the lungs and lymph nodes. The vaginal adenocarcinomas are frequently associated with the more than 1 million American women who were exposed *in utero* to diethylstilbestrol (DES), a synthetic estrogen intended to prevent miscarriage (involuntary loss of the fetus that occurs usually in the first 3 months of pregnancy). DES is known to be a human carcinogen (National Institute of Environmental Health Sciences 2005b).

Approximately 80% of all vaginal cancers are metastatic and treatment options are also complicated by the close proximity of the bladder and the rectum to the vagina (Tewari and DiSaia 2002; Bardawil and Manetta 2006). Removal of the entire vagina (vaginectomy) is often required for survival.

The low incidence of this cancer makes it difficult to evaluate therapies. The Medical University of South Carolina reports that if vaginal cancer is diagnosed early enough, both radical surgery and radiotherapy are curative (Creasman 2005). Adjunctive brachytherapy alone or in conjunction with EBRT is actively used to treat squamous cell carcinomas, adenocarcinomas, melanomas, and small-cell tumors of the vagina (Stryker 2000; Kucera et al. 2001; Tewari et. al. 2001; Tewari and DiSaia 2002; Kushner et al. 2003). All in all these groups achieved 5-year survival rates of 41% to 78% depending primarily on the stage of the disease and except for Stryker, showed no dependence on the cancer's histology.

A retrospective analysis of various radioisotopes and dose rates concluded that neither source nor dose correlates with survival rates although higher dose rates promote more serious late complications when all stages of vaginal cancer are treated with cesium-137, cobalt-60, or iridium-192 brachytherapy and EBRT (Rutowski et al. 2002). The equally detailed retrospective radiotherapy studies by the Washington University in Saint Louis, Missouri suggest that radiation provides very little if any control over distant metastasis (Perez et al. 1988; 1989).

The Texas M. D. Anderson Cancer Center reported that 193 patients encompassing all four stages of squamous cell carcinoma of the vagina were treated with brachytherapy and EBRT to achieve the following 5-year disease free rates: 85% for stage I (tumor limited to the vaginal wall); 78% for stage II (tumor deeper in the vaginal wall and not yet reaching the pelvic wall); 58% for stage III (carcinoma in the pelvic wall) to stage IV (other organs involved). Treatment failure was tumor recurrence in 68%

of stage I and II and 83% in stage III and IV (Frank et al. 2005).

Vulvar Cancer

Cancer of the vulva is considered a rare gynecological malignancy that is typically a squamous cell carcinoma and often associated with prior exposure to the HPV. Most cases involve the large outer lips of the vulva called the labia majora and very rarely the clitoris (erectile tissue having no reproductive function). This cancer is most common in postmenopausal women over 50 although it is has become more prevalent in women in their forties especially those women vulnerable to sexually transmitted diseases.

Vulvar cancer is considered highly curable with 5-year survival rates as high as 98% especially if detected early. The 5-year survival rate reduces to 50% when the cancer has metastasized to the lymph nodes in the groin.

Treatment options have progressed from the surgical removal of the entire vulva (vulvectomy) to more localized surgery especially with evidence that local recurrence is about 10% for both choices (Hacker 1998). In advance stages, postoperative irradiation of the pelvis and groin is often implemented to address the reduction in survival associated with lymph node involvement and recurrence (Perez et al. 1998 of the Washington University Medical Center, Missouri; Katz et al. 2003 of the M. D. Anderson Cancer Center, Texas).

Neoadjuvant radiotherapy (treatment given prior to another therapy) reduces tumor size prior surgery especially when the tumor has grown close to the urethra or anus. But because the vulva is thin and very sensitive, extreme care must be given when implementing radiotherapy to avoid destroying skin cells, or worse, causing necrosis—localized death of tissue. In one case, a

74-year old Japanese woman with stage III cancer first treated with EBRT followed by high-dose interstitial brachytherapy later required a vulvectomy and surgical reconstruction just to preserve the functionality of her anus and ureter (the tube that connects the kidneys to the urinary bladder) (Yamada et al. 2000).

Survival is in fact so dismal for women with recurring incidences of vulvar cancer that in those situations a group in Italy recommends treatment with 30 Gy to 70 Gy radiotherapy plus chemotherapy to achieve 20% 5-year overall survival (Raffetto et al. 2003). Even then it should be recognized that combinations of chemotherapy, radiotherapy, and surgery are generally more risky for the already weakened cancer patient as tissue morbidity increases with each treatment and side effects become more debilitating—a disconcerting result to say the least.

Real or Not

The odds of surviving a genital cancer favor the male of the species. Prostate cancer, the most prevalent cancer in men, has almost no mortality within its first 5 years of being diagnosed as does the significantly rarer testicular cancer (table 7.3) even with metastasis. However, there is serious concern that the near 100% survival reported for men with prostate cancer in the United States, is simply a result of "stage shifting." Stage-shifting simply means that more cancers are detected at an earlier clinically localized stage of development and thus the patient only appears to live longer:

> Higher survival rates do not always result in lower cancer mortality rates; living longer with cancer might reflect how early the cancer was diagnosed rather than an improvement in outcome. (Centers for Disease Control and Prevention 2004a)

Table 7.3

Five-year survival rates and
preferred treatment for cancers of the genitalia

Cancer	Survival Rates (%)	Preferred Treatment
Cervix uteri	92 (local) 56 (regional) 15 (late)	Surgery (local + regional) Chemoradiotherapy (late)
Corpus uteri	96 (local) 67 (regional) 23 (late)	Surgery
Ovary	93 (local) 69 (regional) 30 (late)	Surgery (local + regional) Surgery + Chemotherapy (late)
Penis	68 (all)	Surgery
Prostate	100 (local + regional) 33 (late)	Surgery or Watchful Waiting
Testis	100 (local) 96 (regional) 70 (late)	Surgery + Radiotherapy or Chemotherapy
Vagina	50 (all)	Surgery or Radiotherapy
Vulva	78 (all)	Surgery + Radiotherapy

Note: Survival Rates are 5-year relative survival rates (ratio of the proportion of cancer survivors to the proportion of expected survivors) taken from Ries et al. (2006). Preferred Treatment is intended for informational purposes only, is not intended to constitute medical advice, and should not be relied upon in any such regard. Rates and treatment are not stage specific unless otherwise designated as: (local) cancer confined to the organ itself; (regional) cancer extending no further than surrounding tissue; and (late) cancer has metastasized to distant organs.

Even if prostate cancer is overly diagnosed, stage shifting cannot explain the 100% 5-year survivability of early diagnosed cancer of the testis, which unlike prostate cancer, has no screening methodology.

Vaginal cancer is an example where treatment choices are more complicated because the tumor is in close proximity to vital organs. Medical practitioners are then forced to resort to a second line of defense that includes radiotherapy and chemotherapy. In general, these become treatments of the last resort. The poorer the prognosis, the more likely they will be implemented. In any event, the message is that if an early tumor can be removed surgically then the patient will have the best outcome.

Urinary System Cancers

The urinary system shares some of the same organs as the genital system and unfortunately also its propensity for tumor development. Its function is to filter the blood and in so doing make urine—on average, adults produce nearly 2 quarts of urine per day.

Urine is the magical liquid waste product of the body produced by the kidneys and stored in the urinary bladder until disposed of through the urethra. The bladder can hold roughly ½ quart of urine—a chemical hodge podge of urea (a waste product of digestion), salt, proteins, vitamins, and other chemicals. Urine is 95% water and yet amazingly antibacterial, antiprotozoal, antifungal, and even antiviral. Virtually odorless and colorless, an excess of vitamin B_2 (riboflavin) turns urine a bright yellow, while eating asparagus can give it a distinctive smell.

There are approximately 357,000 cases of bladder cancer and 208,000 cases of kidney cancer annually diagnosed worldwide. Bladder cancer affects 3.3 times more men than women while kidney cancer is 60% more prevalent in males (Mackay et al. 2006). Obesity is a risk factor for kidney cancer and smoking is casually related to bladder cancer (Danaei et al. 2005).

Table 8.1 shows that cancers of the bladder and kidney are surprisingly 1½ more prevalent in the United States and Canada than Japan and the U.K.

Table 8.1

New cases of urinary tract cancers annually diagnosed
per 100,000 population

Cancer	U.S.	Canada	Japan	U.K.
Bladder	20.6	19.3	(11.8)	12.3
Kidney	13.1	13.9	(8.1)	9.1
Ureter	0.8	-	-	-

Source: Jemal et al. (2006); Canadian Cancer Society (2006); National Cancer Center (2005); Cancer Research UK (2002); U.S. Central Intelligence Agency (2006).

Note: In Japan and the U.K., the kidney and the ureter are combined. Rates are age-adjusted and (crude).

Cancer of the bladder is deadlier than cancer of the kidney, killing 135,000 men and 58,000 women annually worldwide (World Health Organization 2005a). In the countries followed (table 8.2) the mortality rates for urinary tract cancers are more or less the same.

Table 8.2

Yearly deaths from urinary tract cancers
per 100,000 population

Cancer	U.S.	Canada	Japan	U.K.
Bladder	4.4	5.1	(4.2)	5.1
Kidney	4.3	4.7	(3.5)	4.5
Ureter	0.3	-	(0.7)	-

Source: Jemal et al. (2006); Canadian Cancer Society (2006); National Cancer Center (2005); Cancer Research UK (2002); U.S. Central Intelligence Agency (2006).

Note: Rates are age-adjusted and (crude).

Adrenal Gland Cancer

The orange-colored adrenal gland is located atop each kidney and divided into an outer and an inner gland that act as two functionally separate organs. The outer part, called the adrenal cortex, produces 2 to 3 dozen different steroid hormones that regulate the sodium-potassium balance in the body, assist in metabolism, and act as anti-inflammatory agents. The inner portion of the adrenal gland is called the adrenal medulla. It produces adrenaline—a hormone that aids in stress release by increasing heart rate and metabolism, constricting the blood vessels, dilating the pupils, and generally preparing the body for the classic flight-or-fight response.

Cancer of the adrenal cortex also called adrenocortical carcinoma is extremely rare, affecting around 200 people per year in the United States. It has no racial predilection and most commonly strikes children in the first decade of life or adults 40 to 60 years of age (Cirillo 2005). The cancer is extremely aggressive and according to work published in Germany, stage I (tumors 2-in and smaller) to stage III (tumors any size that have grown into nearby tissue spreading no further than nearby lymph nodes) are removed by surgery (Allolio and Fassnacht 2006), whereas stage IV (distant metastases) malignancies are treated with chemotherapy (Koschker et al. 2006).

Cancer of the adrenal medulla also called pheochromocytoma is another extremely rare disease. In the United States and throughout the world, the true incidence is unknown. The disease occurs mostly in 20 to 40 year old adults, shows no preference for sex or race, and when infrequently found in children it is almost always inherited (Krishnan and Shirkhoda 2005).

This cancer is commonly associated with hypertension (high-blood pressure) and so early resection is necessary to avoid further complications according to the Texas M. D.

Anderson Cancer Center adding that radiotherapy is best used for palliation since there is no known cure for metastatic or recurrent disease (Pederson and Lee 2003).

Bladder Cancer

Cancer of the urinary bladder can be diagnosed with >90% accuracy using a cystoscope (a flexible lighted telescope inserted through the urethra) for visual examination and biopsy. A cystoscopy does require local anesthesia if done in a physicians office, or sedation if done as an outpatient procedure. When cystoscopy is combined with a newly developed protein specific urine test, the Texas M. D. Anderson Cancer Center claims that bladder cancer can be detected with 99% accuracy (Grossman et al. 2006). However, approximately 5% of all people stricken with this disease have metastasis at the time of diagnosis (Steinberg et al. 2005).

Because the bladder is essentially just a muscular hollow sac, early stage cancer is treated with surgery—a partial cystectomy in which a tumor that does not extend into the surrounding muscle is removed. A radical cystectomy (complete removal of the bladder. plus adjacent organs as needed) results in 75% to 80% long-term, disease-free survival (Dinney 2006). And while this procedure is also the "gold standard" of treatment for tumors that invade the surrounding muscle, within 5 years of treatment close to 50% of those treated will develop metastatic disease (Garcia and Dreicer 2005). Treating invasive bladder cancer with adjuvant chemotherapy can garner a small benefit provided great care is utilized in selecting patients who have both a high risk for recurring disease and an ability to tolerate such therapy (Dinney 2006).

A Harvard Medical School study of 106 invasive bladder cancer patients treated with chemoradiotherapy between 1986 and 1993 at the Boston Massachusetts General Hospital showed no improvement and 56% 5-year overall survival rates compared to cystectomy (Kachnic et al. 1997). Other randomized clinical trial studies by Shipley and coworkers (1998) of the Massachusetts General Hospital, and by Coppin and others (1996) in Canada, of men and women with tumors in which the cancer had begun to grow into the muscle and beyond the connective tissue layer confirmed this lack of improvement in overall survival for invasive bladder cancer patients who underwent chemoradiotherapy with the radiosensitizer cisplatin.

A British group studied 398 invasive bladder cancer patients treated between 1993 and 1996 comparing radiotherapy without chemotherapy to cystectomy and concluded that

> there is no significant difference in the 5-year survival of patients with invasive bladder cancer treated with either radical radiotherapy or radical cystectomy. All forms of radical treatment for bladder cancer are associated with a significant treatment-associated morbidity and mortality. (Chahal et al. 2003)

Kidney Cancer

The kidneys are the bean-shaped organs that produce and eliminate urine. Luckily, we are all blessed with two kidneys and can function reasonably well with only one. Positioned on both sides of the spine and toward the back of the abdomen, two different cancers can develop here— renal cell carcinoma and renal pelvis carcinoma.

Renal cell carcinoma forms in the lining of the blood filtering tubes of the kidney. Surgery is the only effective treatment for localized tumors although a third of the time the disease is metastatic (Sachdeva et al. 2002). The Memorial Sloan-Kettering reports renal cell carcinoma is highly resistant to both chemotherapy and hormonal agents and requires novel therapies (Patel, Chaganti, and Metzer 2006). Metastatic renal cell carcinoma patients face a dismal prospect of 6 to 12 months of life and at best, 2-year survival rates of 10% to 20% (Campbell, Flanigan, and Clark 2003). In Rome, Italy, Mancuso and Sternberg (2005) have described the use of immunotherapy to treat metastatic renal cell carcinoma noting that this cancer is also refractory (non-responsive) to radiotherapy.

Cancer of the upper urinary tract includes malignancies of the renal pelvis and ureter—the nominal 10-inch long tubes connecting each kidney to the bladder. Renal pelvis carcinoma forms in the center of the kidney. These cancers are relatively rare accounting for 10% of all kidney tumors while ureter cancers are even less common, almost all of which are cancers of the transitional cell—cells that may be stretched without breaking apart. Cancers of the upper urinary tract are treated by nephroureterectomy, the removal of the kidney and its ureter (Bamias et al. 2004).

If the tumor is confined to the ureter, it is possible to remove and preserve the kidney. In stage I and II disease, the cancer is completely inside the kidney and so surgery is quite clean, while in more advanced stages, the removal of surrounding tissue and other organs is required. Complete removal of the kidney is called a nephrectomy and at one time it was the treatment of choice for resectable renal cell carcinoma. More recently, nephron-sparing surgery leaves some working kidney, a procedure that is becoming a "safe and effective alternative to radical nephrectomy," according to the Mayo Clinic (Sengupta and Zinke 2005).

New York's Memorial Sloan-Kettering Cancer Center warns that a large majority of people stricken with upper urinary tract carcinomas have locally advanced tumors at the time a nephroureterectomy is performed (Olgac et al. 2004). Approximately half of all locally advanced stage III upper urinary tract carcinoma patients whose cancer has spread to the layer of fat outside the renal pelvis or into the kidney wall will die from their disease mainly due to the inevitable development of distant metastasis (Bamias et al. 2004). The Massachusetts General Hospital reported an actuarial 39% 5-year overall survival in 31 stage III patients using 46.9 Gy adjuvant radiotherapy with and without cisplatin-based chemotherapy (Czito et al. 2004).

Wilms' Tumor

According to the American Cancer Society (2006e), Wilms' tumor accounts for 6% of all cancers in children in the United States—roughly 500 new cases each year. Also called nephroblastoma, this congenital (present at birth) disease affects African Americans more than Caucasians and Caucasians slightly more than Asian Americans. Breslow and coworkers (1993) reporting from the University of Washington, Seattle, point out that this disease is more common in girls than in boys, has a median age of 38 months, and targets boys 6 months earlier than girls. In almost all cases, Wilms' tumors affect only one kidney.

Both Faria and coworkers (1996) of California's Loma Linda University, and Ghosh, Lundstrom, and Edwards (2002) of the Minnesota Mayo Clinic report that early stages of this disease, in which the cancer is found in one kidney, are favorably treated by surgery and chemotherapy, whereas radiation is used only in advanced stages such as when both kidneys are cancerous or in cases characterized by anaplasia (tumor cells having bizarre cellular features). As example, a German study of 440 Wilms' tumor afflicted boys and girls with a median age of 2.9 years who underwent pre-operative chemotherapy demonstrated a 92% 5-year overall survival rate in children having a favorable histology compared to 49% in those children exhibiting anaplasia (Weirich et al. in 2004).

A Cancerous Retreat

Early diagnosis is critical to surviving urinary tract cancers and the effectiveness of a combination visual-chemical screening methodology for bladder cancer cannot be over emphasized. Table 8.3 shows that once a urinary tract tumor is detected, and if it has not metastasized, surgery is effective and survival is high. In general, radiotherapy is of little value in treating these cancers.

Table 8.3

Five-year survival rates and preferred treatment
for urinary tract cancers

Cancer	Survival Rates (%)	Preferred Treatment
Bladder	94 (local) 46 (regional) 6 (late)	Surgery (local + regional) Surgery + Chemotherapy (late)
Kidney	90 (local) 62 (regional) 10 (late)	Surgery (local + regional) Chemotherapy or Immunotherapy (late)
Ureter	50	Surgery + Radiotherapy or Chemoradiotherapy

Note: Survival Rates are 5-year relative survival rates (ratio of the proportion of cancer survivors to the proportion of expected survivors) taken from Ries et al. (2006). Preferred Treatment is intended for informational purposes only, is not intended to constitute medical advice, and should not be relied upon in any such regard. Rates and treatment are not stage specific unless otherwise designated as: (local) cancer confined to the organ itself; (regional) cancer extending no further than surrounding tissue; and (late) cancer has metastasized to distant organs.

There are few certainties in life and tumor regression is not one of them. Renal cell carcinoma, however, is one of few cancers that can spontaneously regress. There are at least 100 documented cases of tumor regression in the literature since 1928 and in one of the more interesting cases, a research group in Iceland collaborating with a Brigham and Women's Hospital researcher in Boston published a paper in 2002 reporting the spontaneous total regression of metastatic renal cell carcinoma in a 47 year old man, who at the time of diagnosis was found to have a 2-inch diameter metastatic tumor in his right lung. The man's infected kidney was surgically removed along with its 19 cubic inch primary tumor. Miraculously, four months later the man's lung tumor disappeared altogether and even more remarkably, he lived disease-free for 9 more years (Thoroddsen et al. 2002).

Chest and Abdomen Cancers

The chest, also called the thorax, extends from the neck to just below the lungs and above the abdomen. It is the part of the body protected by the ribcage. In both sexes, the chest has mammary glands, a pair of sweat glands that in childbearing females produce milk for nourishment and antibodies for immunity. These exocrine glands, so called because they secrete through ducts that develop around the nipple, are supported by the surrounding muscle. Males rarely have sizeable breasts whereas the size and shape in women is highly varied. Moreover, breast asymmetry is common.

Lung cancer is the most frequently occurring cancer in the world and today no one disputes that smoking tobacco is the etiologic (causal) carcinogen in 80% to 90% of all lung cancer (Gezairy 2004). All smoke is fine particles suspended in air and as such it is an irritant when inhaled, and in that sense, marijuana smoke is no less carcinogenic than tobacco smoke. "There is no doubt that marijuana smoke contains carcinogens" (Hollister 1998).

Breast cancer, the second most prevalent cancer in the world with almost 1.2 million new cases per year is almost nonexistent in China and India (Mackay et al. 2006). In the four countries followed here, except for Canada, it is the most prevalent cancer (table 9.1). Tung and coworkers (1999) correlate the lower incidence of breast cancer in Japan, with having children before the age of 30, not being obese, and the later onset of menarche (menstruation.)

Table 9.1

New cases of cancer of the chest and abdomen
annually diagnosed per 100,000 population

Cancer	U.S.	Canada	Japan	U.K.
Breast	72.0	67.4	46.4	61.3
Lung	58.6	68.6	36.8	48.0

Source: Jemal et al. (2006); Canadian Cancer Society (2006); National Cancer Center (2005); Cancer Research UK (2002); U.S. Central Intelligence Agency (2006).
Note: Rates are age-adjusted.

Cancer of the lung and bronchus kills more than 1.3 million people per year—957,000 men and 382,000 women, 97% of whom are 45 years and older at the time of death (World Health Organization 2005a). Lung cancer is a disease in which smoking is not the only risk. The U.S. government calls radon, a product of naturally occurring uranium, the second leading cause of lung cancer, and its Environmental Protection Agency (2005) estimates that radon-222 kills some 21,000 people annually in the United States alone. Because radon is roughly eight times heavier than air it has a tendency to remain in the lungs after exhalation where it prolongs exposure of lung cells to deadly alpha rays.

Breast cancer kills more women than any other form of the disease, 499,000 women annually worldwide (World Health Organization 2005a). It also claims the lives of

3000 men per year. Table 9.2 shows that in the United States, Canada, and the U.K., breast cancer is far less deadly than lung cancer. The disease, in fact, is even less deadly in Japan with Japanese migrants living in the United States or U.K. more at risk than if they lived in their homeland.

Table 9.2

Yearly deaths from cancer of the chest and abdomen
per 100,000 population

Cancer	U.S.	Canada	Japan	U.K.
Breast	13.9	16.0	10.9	15.6
Lung	54.5	58.3	28.1	40.1

Source: Jemal et al. (2006); Canadian Cancer Society (2006); National Cancer Center (2005); Cancer Research UK (2002); U.S. Central Intelligence Agency (2006).
Note: Rates are age-adjusted.

Breast Cancer

Age is the biggest risk factor for breast cancer. In the United States, the likelihood of developing breast cancer grows from less than 0.5% in a 39 year old and younger female to more than 7% in a 70 year old and older woman. Approximately one out of every nine American women will develop breast cancer with Caucasians most likely to get it and African Americans most likely to die from it (Jemal et al. 2006). A retrospective analysis of over 1 million American women by the University of California, San Francisco demonstrated that blacks have higher-grade tumors than whites independent of any screening discrepancy (Smith-Bindman et al. 2006).

Approximately 80% of all breast malignancies are located in the ducts that traverse from the lobules (milk glands) to the nipples, while 10% to 15% of tumors are in the lobules themselves. Breast cancer almost always develops in just one breast and no one side is favored over another. Larger breasts are no more likely to develop cancer than smaller breasts and there is no correlation with the size or shape of the breast, both of which are highly varied in females of all races. The British have found from a study of 252 women some dependence on breast asymmetry—each 3.38-ounce difference in breast mass accounting for a 50% increase in risk of cancer (Scutt, Lancaster, and Manning 2006).

The incidence of breast cancer in men is more than one hundred times less so than in women. Men with breast cancer are typically diagnosed 5 years later than women, and as such, are more likely to be at an advanced stage. The Texas M. D. Anderson Cancer Center suggests that this alone probably accounts for men having an even higher mortality rate than women (Giordano, Buzdar, and Hortobagyi 2002).

The conventional treatments implemented to minimize the frighteningly high mortality in women and men, include surgery, chemotherapy, radiotherapy, and hormonal therapy. The clinical outcome is the same in both sexes. Most breast cancer patients undergo surgery which includes breast-conserving surgery such as lumpectomy (the removal of the cancerous tumor itself including some of the surrounding tissue) and various degrees of mastectomy ranging from the removal of part of the breast containing the cancerous tissue to removal of the entire breast, the muscles of the chest wall, and all of the lymph nodes under the arm.

Adjuvant therapy, here, refers to any combination of chemotherapy, hormonal therapy, and radiotherapy along with surgery, and is often implemented especially when the cancer is no longer confined to the breast and lymph nodes under the arm. Typically radiotherapy is used post-operatively due to the inherent risk of induced damage to the blood supply. The University of California, Irvine points out that when radiotherapy is pre-operatively employed it increases the risk of necrosis (Tewari and DiSaia 2002).

Breast cancer that is classified as "early stage"—no extension of the cancer to the chest walls or outside the chest area—is typically treated with breast-conserving surgery plus EBRT, mastectomy plus reconstruction, or mastectomy alone. Ironically, while the survival of any of these procedures is equivalent, the U.S. government added that one of the risk factors for getting breast cancer in the first place is "treatment with radiation therapy to the breast/chest" (National Cancer Institute 2005b).

Although a lower mortality rate is not achieved through radiotherapy, a short-term gain of reduced tumor size has been measured. For example, one giant meta-analysis of 20,000 women from 1945 to 1985 compared surgery alone to surgery with radiation showing that while tumor recurrence was reduced for both therapies, adjuvant radiotherapy lowered breast cancer mortality by 13% whereas death from other causes actually increased by 21% (Early Breast Cancer Trialists' Collaborative Group 2000).

An American study of 818 women showed that when lumpectomy is coupled with 60 Gy radiotherapy, the size of the tumor is reduced more so than with lumpectomy alone (Fisher et al. 1998). However, once again the addition of radiation did not improve mortality rates. A follow-up study of 1851 women by the same group was still unable to demonstrate an improvement in overall mortality rates with the addition of radiotherapy (Fisher et al. 2002).

In a much broader study of 1973 Italian women with breast cancer who were treated with radical mastectomy (removal of the entire breast, chest muscles and armpit lymph nodes) or partial mastectomy (removal of the tumor and some surrounding tissue) were compared with those who underwent lumpectomy coupled with radiotherapy (Veronesi et al. 1995). Although the lowest recurrence of cancerous tumors occurred with the radical mastectomy, the overall survival rates were still identical for all of three treatments.

A retrospective study of 13,199 Australian breast cancer patients who underwent postmastectomy radiotherapy determined after a 10-year follow-up that when radiotherapy was given with the appropriate dose and encompassed an appropriate target volume, a significant 6.4% absolute increase in survival was obtained (Gebski et al. 2006). In evaluating this study, the Duke University Medical Center reminded the medical community of the increased risk of radiation-induced heart disease that may not be evident until at least 20 years after radiotherapy concluding that shorter-term studies may not be able to determine if there is a true overall survival benefit (Prosnitz and Marks 2005). A group in Canada studying 206,523 women under 60 years of age showed a higher risk for fatal heart attacks 10 to 15 years after radiotherapy of the left breast (Paszat et al. 1999). And in Sweden, research showed that of 54,617 women treated with radiotherapy from 1970 to 1985, those with left breast cancer experienced a higher mortality rate than those with right breast cancer (Rutqvist and Johansson 1990). In the United States, the M. D. Anderson Cancer Center published a 10-year median follow-up evaluation of the long-term effects of breast radiotherapy and predicted a 2.4% increase in heart attack risk after chemoradiotherapy (Woodward et al. 2003). Unfortunately, it is not possible to evaluate how the addition of chemotherapy alone contributed to this outcome.

A separation of variables is often problematic in science and Prosnitz and Marks (2005) are quick to note that commonly used breast cancer chemotherapy agents are potentially damaging to the heart, further expressing uncertainty that current radiotherapy is absolutely safe as women with lymph node involvement may be at risk for heart damage when the radiation field is expanded to treat extended tumors.

A review article published by a Swedish group, analyzed 40 scientific papers involving the use of radiotherapy to treat 41,204 breast cancer patients and summed it up best:

> There is moderate evidence that the decrease in non-cancer specific survival is attributed to cardiovascular disease in irradiated patients. (Rutqvist, Rose, and Cavallin-Stahl 2003)

Unless radiotherapy can be implemented such that the all too inevitable harm to healthy tissue is minimized, there will be no improvement in lifespan for breast cancer patients who rely on it for treatment. Scientists, however, do not give up easily and in Sweden, proton beam therapy with its more favorable dose distribution is thought to be a potentially cost effective alternative to radiation therapies that use X-rays and gamma rays for left-sided breast cancer patients in particular (Lundkvist et al. 2005; Bjork-Eriksson and Glimelius 2005).

Lung Cancer

The lung is the center of the respiratory system. The smaller volume lung on the left side has two lobes, whereas the shorter and wider lung on the right side has three lobes. Together this sponge-like pair of organs brings oxygen into the blood and releases carbon dioxide from inside the body via the alveoli, tiny air sacs inside each lung that provide a surface area several times that of the entire body. This perpetual gas exchange between the cells and the outside world requires adults breathe 6 to 10 liters of air per minute while at rest. When exercising, the exchange rate can exceed 100 liters per minute. Air is normally 0.04% carbon dioxide by volume. Exhaled air has a concentration of carbon dioxide above 3% or so at which point it is an asphyxiant—a gas that causes unconsciousness or death by suffocation. As the lungs expand and contract during this exchange, a thin membrane called the pleura protects and cushions the lungs from being banged into the ribs.

Cancer cells are characteristically oxygen deficient. The constant interaction of oxygen-depleted blood with the millions of alveoli may account for lung tissue being the body's primary metastatic site since here, statistically so many more cells are exposed to effects of other cells than anywhere else.

Lung cancer is divided into two types: small cell lung cancer and non-small cell lung cancer (NSCLC) the latter which accounts for 80% of all lung cancer tumors. Staging is more complicated in NSCLC because this form is less aggressive. Stage III NSCLC, for example, may mean that the disease is in lymph nodes away from the affected lung but still on the same side of the chest, or it is in nodes nearest the affected lung and which have spread to the pleura or middle of the chest, or that it extends above either collarbone, or even that there is more than one tumor in an affected lobe or another organ like the heart or windpipe.

An international group of 78 researchers reported that surgery is the treatment of choice for 5-year survival across all stages of NSCLC but that only one in five people have potentially curative resectable tumors. In spite of the poor prognosis for NSCLC patients, this research group concluded from a meta-analysis of 52 randomized clinical trials that cisplatin favored chemotherapy provided a 12% 5-year survival rate when used with surgery and radiotherapy (Non-small Cell Lung Cancer Collaborative Group 1995).

According to the University of Washington in Seattle, controversy exists as to whether adjuvant radiotherapy actually does improve NSCLC survival rates (Vallières 2002). A 1997 study by Sawyer and coworkers of the Mayo Clinic reported on 224 NSCLC patients with stage III tumors and noted that adjuvant post-operative radiotherapy improved the survival rate from 4% to 27% for high risk patients and from 37% to 45% for intermediate risk patients defining risk as the probability of developing local tumor recurrence and/or dying. Another international study based on 2128 NSCLC patients showed a reduction in survival rates from 55% to 48% when radiotherapy was implemented post-operatively (PORT Meta-analysis Trialists Group 1998).

For most NSCLC patients, where the disease is too extensive, or where the patient is too weak and elderly, radiotherapy alone does not improve survival (Noordijk et al. 1988; Gauden, Ramsay, and Tripcony 1995). However, when combined with chemotherapy some gain is realized. A study of 155 men and women with stage III cancers published in 1990 by Dillman and coworkers of the University of California, San Diego showed improvement in survival of 23% after 3 years using chemoradiotherapy. A statistical analysis of individual chemoradiotherapy studies of 9387 NSCLC patients with locally advanced tumors showed a 13% lower risk of death when a radiosensitizer such as cisplatin was used; and a 27% lower risk in patients with metastatic cancers (Non-small Cell Lung Cancer Collaborative Group 1995).

Several other studies throughout the world demonstrate that chemoradiotherapy significantly improves a person's short-term survival. A randomized study in France of 177 patients, for example, determined that 21% 2-year overall survival rate could be achieved in people with non-resectable tumors given 65 Gy combined with cisplatin-based chemotherapy with local control remaining the major problem for success (Le Chevalier et al. 1991). In the Netherlands, Schaake-Koning and coworkers (1992) similarly found in 331 non-resectable patients a 54% 1-year survival and a 16% 3-year survival. In the United States, a group reported a median survival of 13.8 months for 452 men and women with non-resectable tumors (Sause et al. 1995).

Small cell lung cancer is by far the more aggressive form of this disease:

> Without treatment, small cell carcinoma of the lung has the most aggressive clinical course of any type of pulmonary tumor, with median survival from diagnosis of only 2 to 4 months.... Limited-stage disease, median survival of 16 to 24 months with current forms of treatment.... With tumors that have spread beyond the [thorax] survival of 6 to 12 months is reported with currently available therapy. (National Cancer Institute 2006b)

For treatment purposes, small cell lung cancer distinguishes between patients with tumors limited to the thorax (limited stage) and patients with distant metastases (extensive stage). Chemoradiotherapy is really only used to treat limited stage small cell lung cancer patients. A meta-analysis study of 2103 men and women published in 1992 by Pignon and coworkers in France claimed a 14% reduction in overall mortality while another meta-analysis study by Warde and Payne (1992) in Canada showed an improvement in local control of cancerous tumors at risk of increased treatment related deaths. Others have reported an improvement in overall survival with complete remission (no sign of cancer remaining) by exposing the head to radiation—prophylactic brain radiotherapy—to prevent central nervous system (CNS) metastases, a complication that occurs in 60% of the time (Aupérin et al. 1999). In contrast, some groups have observed no such benefit as radiation failed to prevent brain relapse in one-fifth of 94 patients studied (Laukkanen et al. 1988).

An Italian review paper points out that although small cell lung cancer is on the decline there has been no real improvement in treatment since the 1980's. Chemoradiotherapy still cures 10% to 20% while the addition of the prophylactic brain irradiation provides an additional 5% reduction in mortality for limited stage patients. And a little more than half those with extensive disease respond to chemotherapy achieving 20% to 30% complete remission (Rosti et al. 2006).

Small cell lung cancer is also one of the most common causes of superior vena cava syndrome (SVCS), a frightening disease in which the blood supply from the head, neck, and arms is constricted from entering the heart through the large superior vena cava vein. Tumors often enlarge lymph nodes in the chest adjacent to the superior vena cava vein—thin-walled and under pressure—which compresses and causes breathing difficulties and chest pain. SVCS is usually treated with chemotherapy and in those cases where the tumor is insensitive to chemotherapy, Nicholson and coworkers (1997) have demonstrated retrospectively that stents are superior to palliative radiotherapy.

Mesothelioma

Asbestos is a naturally occurring fibrous mineral with fire retardant properties that make it immensely useful as a thermal insulator. Unfortunately, it is also a serious health hazard listed by the National Institute for Occupational Safety and Health as a "potential" carcinogen (Centers for Disease Control and Prevention 2004b). Airborne asbestos has been linked to higher than normal incidences of lung, stomach, and colon cancer, and mesothelioma—a cancer of the mesothelium (a protective lining of the body cavity and many internal organs including the lung). Thus today the industrial use of asbestos is highly regulated and in some countries its use is banned altogether.

Mesothelioma affects some 2000 people per year in the United States, mostly men. Incidence is on the rise with more than 70% of all mesothelioma cancer patients having a history of prior exposure to asbestos according to the Wayne State University in Detroit (Martino and Pass 2004).

Recent studies by Carbone and Rdzanek (2004) in the United States indicate that genetic factors and a Simian virus (pathogen that infects monkeys and other primates) may predispose patients with subsequent asbestos exposure to mesothelioma. This disease manifests itself some 20 years or more after asbestos exposure and has been a rich source of lawsuit revenue. Settlement awards upwards of several million dollars in the United States are not uncommon with 40% or so of any compensation going to the patient's attorney.

Extremely short survival rates of approximately 1 year characterize this disease (de Vries and Long 2003; Villena Garrido et al. 2004). Surgery is the most common treatment for mesothelioma with advanced cases requiring a pneumonectomy (removal of the entire lung). To date no treatment is curative (van Ruth et al. 2003).

Adjuvant chemotherapy coupled with surgery is the most promising option for mesothelioma patients offering 35 months overall survival rates (Aziz, Jilaihawi, and Prakash 2002). The M. D. Anderson Cancer Center in Texas demonstrated 65% 1-year survival rates with IMRT noting side effects that included nausea and breathing difficulties (Ahamad et al. 2003). In cases where surgery is not an option, a University of Chicago experience showed that chemotherapy gave a 1-year overall median survival; not great, but 3 months more than the usual (Vogelzang et al. 2003).

Thymic Carcinoma

The thymus gland is an endocrine gland located at the base of the neck under the sternum (breastbone) and is responsible for manufacturing white blood cells called lymphocytes that are used to fight infection. The thymus provides antibodies and is remarkable in that it actually shrinks with age.

Two types of cancer originate in the thymus gland— thymomas and thymic carcinomas. Both types are quite rare and account for only 0.2% to 1.5% of all malignancies with thymic carcinomas accounting for 0.06% of all thymic tumors. The representative age group diagnosed with these cancers is 40 to 60-year olds, approximately 30% of whom show no symptoms other than a strong cough often confused with bronchitis (inflammation of the bronchus) (National Cancer Institute 2005f). Thymic carcinomas metastasize rapidly whereas thymomas are slow growing, rarely metastasize and are associated with secondary malignances. Thymic cancers are extremely rare; and only 500 to 700 thymomas are annually diagnosed in the United States (American Cancer Society 2006d).

According to the University of California, Davis, complete resection is the standard treatment for early stage thymomas, in which the cancer has not spread beyond the gland, the nearby fatty tissue, or the mediastinum. When the cancer has spread to other tissues or organs, surgery plus radiotherapy is used (Lara 2000). Thymic carcinoma typically has a 38% 5-year overall survival rate with complete resection offering perhaps the best survival. If the thymic carcinoma cannot be completely surgically removed then chemoradiotherapy is implemented, reports one 15-year Japanese study of 40 patients (Ogawa et al. 2002). Cancer of the thymus killed 164 Japanese men and 90 women in 2003 alone (National Cancer Center 2005).

The Preventable Killer

Tumors of the chest and abdomen are in all cases, except small cell lung cancer, effectively removed with surgery if detected early (table 9.3). When this is the case, breast cancer in particular has an impressive 5-year survival rate.   There is concern, however, that like

Table 9.3

Five-year survival rates and preferred treatment for cancers of the chest and abdomen

Cancer	Survival Rates (%)	Preferred Treatment
Breast	98 (local) 83 (regional) 26 (late)	Surgery
Lung (non small cell)	51 (local) 17 (regional) 2 (late)	Surgery (local + regional) Chemoradiotherapy (late)
Lung (small cell)	20 (local) 10 (regional) 2 (late)	Chemoradiotherapy
Mesothelioma	15 (local) 10 (regional) 7 (late)	Surgery (local + regional) Surgery + Chemotherapy (late)
Thymus	61	Surgery (local + regional) Surgery + Chemoradiotherapy (late)

Note: Survival Rates are 5-year relative survival rates (ratio of the proportion of cancer survivors to the proportion of expected survivors) taken from Ries et al. (2006). Preferred Treatment is intended for informational purposes only, is not intended to constitute medical advice, and should not be relied upon in any such regard. Rates and treatment are not stage specific unless otherwise designated as: (local) cancer confined to the organ itself; (regional) cancer extending no further than surrounding tissue; and (late) cancer has metastasized to distant organs.

prostate cancer the survival rate of breast cancer is subject to stage-shifting or other investigator biases (Krzyzanowska and Tannock 2005). Even more unnerving, the 5-year survival rates for breast cancer in the United States may not in fact account for a latent decrease in survival attributed to radiation and chemotherapy treatment-related deaths.

Radiotherapy is used as part of the preferred treatment of late stage lung cancer, a disease with almost no chance of survival (table 9.3). In 2006, Varian Medical Systems, which touts itself as the world's leading manufacturer of medical technology for treating cancer with radiation therapy announced building a 134,000 square foot manufacturing facility in Beijing, China to exploit the country's emerging cancer market–300 million male cigarette smokers equivalent to the entire U.S. population. Business is business and smoking is predicted to kill one third of all Chinese men who are 30 years and younger (World Health Organization 2002).

Head and Neck Cancers

The brain is the center of the central nervous system (CNS)—almost 3 pounds of nerve cells protectively housed in the skull. The thalamus (subdivision of the brain that acts as a relay station for sensory organs), and the hypothalamus-pituitary gland (the controller of heart and respiratory rate, hunger and thirst, as well as body temperature and blood pressure), all share space beneath the convoluted gray matter—two cerebral hemispheres of nerve cells where all thought and memory occur. A passageway at the base of the skull allows for the brain to make a contiguous link to the spinal cord—the so-called "body's information superhighway," a neural network that runs the length of the back and which senses and controls all movement.

Primary cancers of the brain are rare and almost all CNS cancers develop in and around the brain as a result of metastases from other malignancies outside the CNS such as the lung, breast, skin, and kidney. Table 10.1 shows that cancers of the brain occur with essentially the same

Table 10.1

New cases of cancers of the head and neck
diagnosed annually per 100,000 population

Cancer	U.S.	Canada	Japan	U.K.
Brain and CNS	6.3	7.6	(3.3)	6.9
Larynx	3.2	3.5	(2.7)	3.1
Oral cavity	10.4	9.7	(7.2)	6.4
Retinoblastoma	<0.1	-	-	<0.1
Thyroid	10.1	10.3	(6.3)	2.2

Source: Jemal et al. (2006); Canadian Cancer Society (2006);
    National Cancer Center (2005); Cancer Research UK (2002);
    U.S. Central Intelligence Agency (2006).
Note: Rates are age-adjusted and (crude).

frequency in the United States, Canada, and the U.K. and at a rate that is inexplicably twice that of Japan. The table also shows that cancers of the oral cavity (lip, gum, tongue, mouth, and throat or pharynx) are a more commonly diagnosed malignancy. Indeed, oral cavity cancer is the eleventh most prevalent cancer in the world—annually afflicting 176,000 males and 98,000 females (Mackay et al. 2006). Cigarette, cigar, and pipe smoking, tobacco chewing, and heavy drinking (spirits more than beer and wine) are well known risk factors for the development of almost all oral cavity cancers (Castellsague et al. 2004; Danaei et al. 2005). Interestingly enough, none of these cancers are linked to marijuana use (Rosenblatt et al. 2004).

In the four countries followed, cancer of the larynx, an organ of the upper respiratory tract, is about half as common as brain cancer and unequivocally linked with smoking and drinking (Menvielle et al. 2004). Cancer of the larynx is four times more likely in males in the United States, Canada, and the U.K. and fourteen times more prevalent in males in Japan. In contrast, cancer of the thyroid—the large endocrine gland that sits just below the larynx—is three to four times more prevalent in females in all four countries. An American prospective study of 89,835 Canadian women showed that the high incidence of thyroid cancer in Canada was unrelated to alcohol consumption, hormonal factors, menstruation, reproductive factors, or smoking (Navarro Silvera, Miller, and Rohan 2005).

Oral cavity cancers are deadly worldwide. These diseases kill 236,000 men and 106,000 women per year. Less than 10% of the total are 44 years and younger (World Health Organization 2005a). The mortality rates for oral cavity cancers in the United States, Canada, Japan and the U.K. are relatively low (table 10.2) undoubtedly because of the decline in smoking, with Japan, where 51% of the men smoke, thus far being the least successful of the four in discouraging the habit (World Health Organization 2002).

Table 10.2

Yearly deaths from cancers of the head and neck
per 100,000 population

Cancer	U.S.	Canada	Japan	U.K.
Brain and CNS	4.3	5.0	(1.2)	5.0
Eye	<0.1	-	(<0.1)	-
Larynx	1.3	1.5	(0.8)	1.0
Oral cavity	2.5	3.3	(4.1)	2.3
Thyroid	0.5	0.5	1.3	0.4

Source: Jemal et al. (2006); Canadian Cancer Society (2006); National Cancer Center (2005); Cancer Research UK (2002); U.S. Central Intelligence Agency (2006).
Note: Rates are age-adjusted and (crude).

The significantly higher mortality rate for thyroid cancer in Japan compared to the United States, Canada, and the U.K. probably reflects the long-term effect of the Hiroshima and Nagasaki bombings of 1945 on Japanese children, whereas the unusually low mortality rate for brain and CNS cancer in Japan is thought to be due to a loss of patients during follow-up (Kaneko et al. 2002).

Brain Cancer

Brain tumors occur at any age and yet they are the leading cause of death from cancer in persons 35 years and younger and are second only to leukemia as a cause of pediatric cancer in the United States (Huff 2005). Primary cancers of the brain and CNS are especially preventable in that

> the only established environmental risk factor for brain tumors is radiation.... Most radiation-induced brain tumors are caused by radiation to the head given for the treatment of other cancers. (American Cancer Society 2006f)

According to a report from Sweden, using cellular (analogue and digital) and cordless telephones can lead to a two-fold increased risk of developing a malignant brain tumor (Hardell, Cardell, and Mild 2006). However, these devices emit only radio frequency waves that are incapable of causing ionization and so many researchers dispute that a correlation with cancer is possible. Adding to the debate, recent work by Diem and coworkers (2005) in Austria suggests that such low-energy radiation may in fact damage DNA *in vitro*—a controversy for sure in that there is no known causal relationship between non-ionizing radiation and cancer.

Interestingly, when the brain itself is the source of the tumor the cancer rarely spreads to other parts of the body. Nearly half of all primary brain tumors and a quarter of all spinal cord tumors are classified as gliomas. A glioma is a tumor that originates from supporting nerve cells (neurons) and not the neurons involved in signaling and information processing. Different types of glioma include astrocytoma, gliobastoma, and oligodendroglioma.

Surgery is commonly recommended for most brain tumors except for those that are located deep in the brain or when patient's chance of recovery or recurrence is poor. Benign tumors are nearly as harmful as malignant ones when they exert pressure between the brain and the skull. In general, the more incurable or deep-seated the malignant tumors are, the more likely a person with brain cancer will be recommended for radiotherapy or chemotherapy. One obvious concern is the known risk of radiation-induced brain tumors that have been positively associated with radiation dose (Sadetzki et al. 2005).

Certain slow growing tumors labeled as "low-grade" that are common in children are considered treatable by surgery or surgery plus radiotherapy an addition that is considered quite controversial by the University of Virginia in Charlottesville (Lopes and Laws Jr. 2002).

In adult patients, the Mayo Clinic in Minnesota claimed an improvement in over-all survival rates for post-operative EBRT doses equal to or greater than 53 Gy, but in only one particular type of glioma (Shaw et al. 1989). A group in the Netherlands showed no improvement in the survival of 311 adult glioma patients given 54 Gy EBRT after surgery (Karim et al. 2002). At the same time, a Finnish study noted that post-operatively irradiated adults later exhibited long-term cognitive impairment (ability to think, reason, and remember) (Surma-aho et al. 2001). All three findings very clearly highlight the sensitivity of healthy brain tissue to radiation and thus a need for stereotactic radiosurgery (SRS).

Indeed, SRS is a welcome alternative to surgical resection especially when the tumor is inaccessible. Generally, SRS finds application in people 65 years and younger and those with tumors no larger than 1½ inches or so in diameter. In particular, it has proven beneficial to multiple brain metastases patients who account for nearly half of all brain cancer patients (Jawahar and coworkers 2004) of the Louisiana State University Health Sciences Center and even more so when combined with conventional surgical tumor removal (Meier et al. 2004). According to the Mayo Clinic in Minnesota, only four cases of radiation-induced tumors following SRS are known (McIver and Pollock 2004), possibly because most patients with brain cancer do not live long enough for a second malignancy to develop.

In those patients with the more aggressive, incurable brain cancers, often referred to as malignant gliomas, it is difficult to compare treatments as survival is short and controlled experiments are not feasible. Combining surgery with adjuvant chemoradiotherapy shows various degrees of success, increasing overall survival rates for malignant gliomas, but without any knowledge gained as to what might have been the "best" treatment (Chang et al. 1983; Loeffler et al. 1992; Fontanesi et al. 1993; Macdonald, 2001):

> High-grade malignant glioma … have a poor prognosis…. Relapse is nearly universal, responses in recurrent disease are not enduring, and quality of life because of tumor growth is poor. New treatment strategies that address symptom control and quality of life as well as progression-free and overall survival are urgently needed. (Macdonald 2001)

Meningiomas are tumors that originate in the meninges (outer covering of the brain). Like leukemia and thyroid cancer, meningiomas are another disease that have been linked to radiation exposure showing a higher than normal incidence in Hiroshima atomic bomb survivors (Shintani et al. 1999).

According to the University of Utah, meningiomas are the second most common CNS tumor and account for approximately 20% of all such tumors in the United States. These slow growing, mostly benign growths are twice as commonly diagnosed in women between 50 and 60 years, and are typically removed surgically (Ragel and Jensen 2003). If total tumor resection is not possible due to location or the likelihood of recurrence then alternative therapies are required. A British study of 82 people with surgically removed meningiomas followed by EBRT demonstrated an impressive 71% 10-year survival rate (Nutting et al. 1999). Five years later, the UCLA School of Medicine reported that 29 meningioma patients who underwent SRS after conventional surgery showed remarkably, a 100% 3-year overall survival rate (Selch et al. 2004).

Unfortunately, in both sexes equally, some two in 100 meningiomas are malignant, and have a 33% to 78% chance of recurring depending on their histology (Ragel and Jensen 2003). In dealing with this problem, a group in Austria treated 16 primary and recurrent malignant meningioma patients with 40 Gy to 70 Gy EBRT and demonstrated good local tumor control and 87% 5-year survival but only if more than 60 Gy was used (DeVries et al. 1999).

Another part of the brain, the pituitary gland is a pea-sized endocrine gland located at the base of the skull. It is often called the "master gland" because the hormones it secretes affect virtually all of the physiological functions in the body. Pituitary tumors are the most commonly encountered intracranial cancers, accounting for approximately 10% of the total according to Case Western Reserve University and University Hospitals of Cleveland (Arafah and Nasrallah 2001). At all stages, surgery is the treatment of choice and radiotherapy is rarely recommended:

Complications caused by radiation therapy itself are many, and some are serious. One of the serious complications seen in some [pituitary tumor] patients, within a short period of time, is worsening visual symptoms secondary to edema, tumor hemorrhage and optic nerve necrosis. Other complications include increased risk of developing malignant brain tumors, brain necrosis and dementia. (Arafah and Nasrallah 2001)

The closely related hypothalamus gland is located directly above the pituitary gland. It too is an endocrine gland and is somewhat facetiously referred to as the "power behind the throne" because it regulates pituitary hormone secretion. Hypothalamic tumors are typically nonmetastatic gliomas in children, and in contrast, a result of metastasis to the hypothalamus gland in adults. Radiation is both a risk factor and a therapeutic solution for this disease (Jasmin 2004).

Laryngeal Cancer

Laryngeal cancer is the name given to malignancies of the larynx or voice box, a nominal 2-inch by 2-inch organ that sits atop the trachea or windpipe. In adult males, the larynx is a somewhat more prominent lump that is commonly referred to as the Adam's apple. Three carcinomas are known to occur here: glottic carcinoma (60% incidence) involves the vocal cords; supraglottic carcinoma (35% incidence) involves the epiglottis (flap of cartilage protecting the trachea from foods entering it); and subglottic carcinoma (5% incidence) refers to cancer below the vocal cords (American Cancer Society 2005c).

Glottic carcinoma is often curable because the vocal cords are devoid of lymphatics. Cure rates of 75% to 95% are achieved if it has not spread to neighboring lymph nodes and if the patient makes changes in lifestyle (Gowda et al. 2003). Even then, however, glottic carcinoma patients are at high risk for other cancers involving the head and neck and recurrences are common within 3 years of treatment.

Surgery is curative for locally controlled glottic tumors that typically require a laryngectomy (surgical removal of the larynx) although modern techniques allow for removal of only part of the larynx so that normal speech function is preserved. EBRT alone is also useful in preserving a patient's ability to speak (Eksteen et al. 2003). At the same time, a number of other groups have demonstrated that EBRT can preserve an 80% and greater 5-year overall survival rate in circumstances where the cancer is confined to an area just above and below the vocal cords (Gowda et al. 2003; Franchin et al. 2003; Zouhair et al. 2004).

In the more advanced stage III (cancer has grown throughout the larynx and not spread elsewhere) and stage IV (cancer has spread to at least the lymph nodes outside the larynx), Shikama and coworkers (2003) in Japan have demonstrated impressive 58% and 35% 5-year overall survival rates, respectively with preoperative 38 Gy radiotherapy. A group in Spain used cisplatin based chemotherapy with hyperfractionated radiotherapy to further confine the cancer in 73 stage IV patients and achieve 42% 5-year overall survival (de la Vega et al. 2003).

The John Hopkins research group of Forastiere (2003) realized organ preservation while suppressing distant metastases using concomitant application of cisplatin and radiotherapy but not without causing mucositis (an inflammation that manifests itself as mouth sores) and failing to improve survival.

Beginning in 2004, a number of groups including Eisbruch and coworkers in the United States and Clark and coworkers in the U.K. reported the potential of IMRT to treat advanced glottic cancer patients without damaging the spinal cord. These studies emphasized the need for local tumor control but did not provide anything more than an actuarial survival benefit:

> No randomized trial has yet been conducted to show [IMRT] superiority over conventional treatments, and only a few meaningful retrospective studies are available that show its potential and its possible drawbacks. (Grégoire and Maingon 2004)

Furthermore, the Belgian scientists Verellen and Vanhavere reported as far back as 1999 that IMRT yielded "an increase in the risk for secondary malignancies with a factor 8" that they attributed to the larger volume of normal tissue that is necessarily irradiated when the IMRT dose is maximized to destroying the laryngeal tumor.

Supraglottic cancer has poor prognosis as a result of the abundant source of lymphatic drainage in this area and thus 25% to 50% of those diagnosed present with lymph node involvement (Sonne and Schaefer 2003).   A retrospective study of 653 superglottic laryngeal patients evaluated nine different treatments and concluded that surgery with or without adjuvant radiotherapy did not give a survival advantage because of recurrence and distant metastasis (Sessions, Lenox, and Spector 2005).

Ophthalmic Cancers

Cancer shows no mercy and when it strikes the eye, the loss of sight is but one of its casualties. Uveal melanoma also called intraocular melanoma is a malignancy of the middle eye and the most common cancer of the eye with an annual incidence that varies with race/ethnicity: 0.31 (black), 0.38 (Asian), 1.67 (Hispanic), 6.02 (non-Hispanic white) per million people in the United

States; white Americans are eighteen-times more likely to develop this cancer than black Americans (Hu et al. 2005).

At least 30% of all people with cancer of the eye develop systemic metastasis, occurring usually in the liver. Consequently, 5-year, 15-year, and 25-year mortality rates of 62%, 90%, and 98% respectively, after cancer diagnosis are representative (Kujala, Makatie, and Kivela 2003).

Ophthalmic tumors are often treated with radioactive disks called plaques that are surgically attached to the surface of the eye. A gold casing is often employed to house the radioisotope so that the radiation is directed into the eye and not away from it. A study of 65 French patients treated with cobalt-60 and ruthenium-106 plaques gave an impressive disease free survival rates of 83% and 74% after 5 years and 10 years respectively (Bacin et al. 1998). Similar success was also achieved with palladium-103 plaques by Finger and coworkers (2002) at Saint Vincent's Comprehensive Cancer Center in New York City and with iodine-125 plaques by Quivey and coworkers (1993) at the University of California, San Francisco.

Irrespective of which radioisotope is used in treatment, the Thomas Jefferson University in Philadelphia, found that plaque therapy is often associated with reduced visual acuity ranging from 20/200 to no light perception adding that the problem was observed in some 68% of the 10-year follow up patients monitored (Shields et al. 2000).

More recently linac-based SRS in combination with IMRT has been used to treat uveal melanoma in 40 people, but the report failed to provide statistics supporting the advantage of IMRT (Georg et al. 2003).

Choroidal melanoma is a uveal melanoma tumor located in the blood-rich region behind the retina (the light sensitive back of the eyeball). If diagnosed before it has had opportunity to metastasize to the liver, its primary target, it is treated with some success by ophthalmic plaque therapy in combination with EBRT:

Unfortunately, after all forms of radiotherapy ... an average of 16.3% of patients treated with radiotherapy subsequently require enucleation [surgical removal of the eyeball] because of tumor regrowth or uncontrollable neovascular glaucoma [build-up of pressure within the eyeball]. (Finger 1997)

In a 2003 paper, Straatsma of the UCLA Medical Center reported that 1317 choroidal melanoma patients treated with iodine-125 plaque radiotherapy showed a 5-year overall mortality of 18% compared to 30% in 1003 people who received no treatment.

A year later a group in France reported that 213 men and women plagued with small to medium sized ophthalmic tumors and treated with ruthenium-106 plaque radiotherapy experienced 5-year and 10-year survival rates of 82% and 72%, respectively, noting, however, all too common incidences of local recurrence (16%) and enucleation (18%) (Rouberol et al. 2004).

A retrospective study by Harvard University of 76 eyes in 63 choroidal metastatic cancer patients treated with proton beam therapy between 1989 and 2000 justifiably boasted 84% regression 5 months after treatment and no need for enucleation. Minor complications such as madarosis (eyelash loss), glaucoma, and cataract (clouding of the eye lens) were noted in 56% of the cases (Tsina et al. 2005)—an acceptable price for anyone threatened with blindness and death.

Oral Cavity Cancers

Almost all malignancies of the oral cavity are squamous cell carcinomas, which like melanomas, are more commonly found in light skinned people exposed to intense sunlight. Squamous cell carcinomas of the lip are significantly less prevalent in women, a benefit that has been ascribed by the University of Southern California to the sunscreening effect of lipstick (Pogoda and Preston-Martin 1996).

A massive retrospective study of 11,666 men and 5717 women in Finland from 1953 to 1999 concluded that

> the incidence of lip cancer decreased in males, probably because of a decrease in smoking and in outdoor work. The incidence of intra-oral cancers increased in both genders, possibly because of increased alcohol consumption. (Tarvainen et al. 2004)

Squamous cell lip cancer of all stages is effectively treated with radiation. An Italian group reports that 62 Gy brachytherapy yields actuarial 5-year and 10-year overall survival rates of 76% and 53%, respectively with patients reporting a satisfactory cosmetic outcome (Tombolini et al. 1998). A German group treated squamous cell carcinomas of the lip and adjacent organs in 201 patients using adjuvant brachytherapy in combination with EBRT claiming 64% 5-year overall survival for stage I (localized 1-inch or smaller tumor) and II (localized 2-inch or smaller tumor) and 39% 5-year overall survival for stage III (cancer spread to an adjacent lymph node) and IV (cancer spread to more than one lymph node) with most failures due to local recurrence (Grabenbauer et al. 2001). Lastly, a French group realized 5-year overall survival rates of 70% in stage I and II, 44% in stage III, and 22% in stage IV, concluding that brachytherapy alone was better when the cancer was localized in terms of overall survival and radiation-induced tissue damage (Lapeyre et al. 2004).

Cancer of the oropharynx includes malignancies of the soft palate (back of the mouth) and tonsils (lymph tissue on both sides of the mouth). The tonsils are two non-essential glands located at the back of the throat and which effectively disappear by adolescence. Tonsillar carcinoma, the most prevalent oropharyngeal carcinoma, has the strongest association with HPV of any nongenital cancer according to a Finnish publication. And while it is not sexually transmitted, "husbands of patients with HPV associated cervical cancer had an increased risk of tonsillar cancer" (Syrjänen 2004).

Oropharyngeal cancers are treated with surgery, radiotherapy, and chemotherapy depending on the extent of the growth and receptiveness of the tumor. Clinical trials of stage I to IV cancers treated with adjuvant chemotherapy showed 5-year overall survival rates of 67% to 77% compared to 46% for surgery alone (Kovacs et al. 2003; Kovacs 2004). Groups in Taiwan and France reported a further improvement with chemoradiotherapy, but with more severe side effects than with radiotherapy alone (Lin et al. 2003; Denis et al. 2004). Liu and coworkers (2003) in Taiwan added that introducing IMRT further reduced mortality rates and gave 82% 3-year overall survival rates independent of stage, failing, however, to retard distant metastasis. According to a Swiss group, some side effects associated with treating this cancer with radiotherapy include trouble swallowing, xerostomia (dry mouth), sticky saliva, and difficulties in eating in social settings (Tschudi, Stoeckli, and Schmid 2003).

Cancer of the nasopharynx (upper part of the throat behind the nose) was successfully treated with 70 Gy chemoradiotherapy at the University of Chicago between 1990 and 1999 achieving 77% 5-year overall survival rates in 27 stage III and IV patients 33% of whom experienced acute toxicity (Oh et al. 2003). Three years after this work was published, the Memorial Sloan-Kettering Cancer Center reported using IMRT with concurrent chemotherapy realizing in 69 stage III and IV patients, 83% 3-year overall survival with a lower incidence of xerostomia (Wolden et al. 2006).

Cancer of the hypopharynx (deepest part of the throat) affects approximately 2770 Americans annually (American

Cancer Society 2005c). Hypopharyngeal tumors are usually diagnosed at an advanced stage with the patient already showing distant metastases and other primary tumors. A 7-year Japanese retrospective study of 74 patients with squamous cell carcinoma of the hypopharynx noted a 21-month mean survival adding that surgery is "unnecessary" for locoregional tumor control (Tateda 2005). However, if this cancer is diagnosed early enough, another Japanese group analyzing the use of surgery and adjuvant radiotherapy to treat stage I and II claimed a 66% 5-year overall survival rate (Nakamura et al. 2006).

The tongue provides us with the ability to taste, chew, swallow, and speak. It is not an organ that we can easily do without. The part of the tongue that sticks out, so to speak, is called the oral tongue. Small conspicuous tumors on its sides are often surgically removed or treated with EBRT followed by a brachytherapy boost. According to work in Japan, a large tumor size accompanied by ulceration is used to predict prognosis and the probability of lymph node metastasis whereby survival is reduced (Yamazaki et al. 2004).

In treating stage I (T1 size lesion) and stage II (T2 size lesion) cancers of the tongue that have not spread to the lymph nodes, the choice between surgery and radiotherapy is mainly based on cosmetics, functionality, and the expertise of the caregivers to provide an overall cure rate of 90% to 100%. Stage III cancers involve the lymph nodes or larger lesions and stage IV tumors have spread to more than one lymph node or another organ. These cancers are more likely to require a combination of surgery and radiotherapy as the risk of distant metastases reduces the 5-year overall survival rate to as low as 22% (Po Wing Yuen et al. 2002).

In 1992, Pernot and coworkers reported from France that 76 Gy interstitial brachytherapy using iridium-192 alone gave better local tumor control than when it was combined with EBRT.   Ten years later, the Washington University School of Medicine in Saint Louis, Missouri published a retrospective study showing that 332 oral tongue cancer patients treated between 1957 and 1996 in the United States had a 73% 5-year overall disease-specific survival if treated by surgery compared to 46% with radiotherapy. However, the best results for late stage cancer patients were achieved with a combination of surgery and radiotherapy; less than half of the 332 treated died from their tumor and 21% developed secondary tumors that killed slightly more than the remaining half (Sessions et al. 2002).

Cancer of the base of the tongue is usually more advanced when diagnosed at which time metastasis is in progress and prognosis is poor. In 2003, Sessions and coworkers published a retrospective study of 262 men and women treated between 1955 and 1998 in the United States that demonstrated a 5-year overall disease-specific survival of 70% with local resection compared to 40% with radiotherapy.   The combination of local resection and radiation resulted in 50% overall survival and radiotherapy clearly did benefit the ability of the person to speak and to swallow.   Nonetheless,   the   prognosis   remains disheartening:

> Cancer of the base of tongue is a lethal disease, and its treatment results in significant disability. No treatment produced a significantly improved survival advantage. (Sessions et al. 2003)

Parathyroid Cancer

There are four or more parathyroid glands, all located adjacent the thyroid gland.   These endocrine glands produce the parathyroid hormone that regulates the use and storage of calcium in the blood. The concentration of calcium is critical as it is associated with muscle contraction, bone strength, and neural response.

Cancer of the parathyroid glands is extremely rare with less 100 cases annually diagnosed in the United States. If confined to an individual gland surgery is extremely effective as the tumors are slow growing and usually detected early due to symptoms associated with the over-production of calcium. Because benign tumors exhibit similar symptoms and only 0.017% of parathyroid tumors causing the over production of calcium are cancerous, the Hospital of the University of Pennsylvania, Philadelphia states that it is not uncommon for this cancer to be undetected until the tumor has been surgically removed. Moreover,

> aggressive surgical resection with en bloc removal of any adjacent invading structures is the best chance for cure leading to a 10-year survival rates of 49%. (Fraker 2000)

Based on relatively small patient populations, the Mayo Clinic in Rochester, Minnesota (Munson et al. 2003) and the University of Texas M. D. Anderson Cancer Center in Houston (Clayman, Gonzalez, and El-Naggar 2004) published convincing retrospective studies that found adjuvant post-operative radiotherapy minimized local tumor recurrence. The Texas group claimed 5-year and 10-year survival rates of 85% and 77%, respectively for this disease.

Retinoblastoma

Retinoblastoma is a rare pediatric disease of the retina and yet it is one of the most common eye tumors found in children. It was the first childhood cancer linked to a genetic defect and the gene identified is the first known tumor suppressor for human cancer according to Deegan (2003) of the Georgetown University School of Medicine.

Retinoblastoma affects some 300 children annually in the United States, primarily infants and 95% of the cases are in children younger than 5 years old. Boys and girls of all races are equally victimized. If the cancer is found in one eye only (unilateral retinoblastoma) it tends to affect older children and is generally not considered hereditary. If the cancer is found in both eyes (bilateral retinoblastoma) it is most definitely hereditary, likely to recur (Ries et al. 1999), and commonly associated with tumors in the brain at which point the disease is no longer curable

Typical treatment regiments for retinoblastoma include rigorous chemotherapy to reduce the tumor size followed by surgery with a greater than 90% cure rate in the United States and the U.K. In developing countries such as India, most children with retinoblastoma will die. Radiotherapy is generally avoided as the chance of incurring additional tumors including sarcoma increases with radiation dose and is highest among children who undergo treatment early and are saddled with a genetic predisposition to this disease (Wong et al. 1997; Garwicz et al. 2000; Watts 2003).

Those children with localized tumors and little hope of keeping their vision will typically undergo enucleation. Children with more extensive tumors but with a reasonable chance of maintaining their vision are likely to undergo chemotherapy which unfortunately is often associated with tumor recurrences that necessitate further treatment—a *Sophie's Choice* for the children's parents and their doctor:

> Creating false hope and the need for enucleation after months of chemotherapy and multiple trips to the operating room can be extremely distressing to all parties involved. (Deegan 2003)

If the tumors recur or become metastatic, more desperate measures are required, such as intravenous chemoreduction (locally injecting chemotherapeutic agents into the tumor), laser photocoagulation (cauterizing blood vessels to the tumor with a laser), thermotherapy (destroying the tumor with a laser), cryotherapy (destroying the tumor by freezing it with liquid nitrogen), EBRT, and iodine-125 plaque radiotherapy (Ocular Oncology Service 2005). A comparison was made of these methods by the Thomas Jefferson University in Philadelphia, Pennsylvania which concluded that in 141 children treated from 1976 to 1999, plaque radiotherapy provided the best treatment— 79% tumor control 5 years post-therapy—but not without introducing a number of radiation complications: cataracts in 31%, glaucoma in 11%, and various incidences of blurred vision associated with retinal damage (Shields et al. 2000).

The Saint Jude Children's Research Hospital in Memphis, Tennessee claimed success in obtaining disease-free survival in four metastatic (bone and bone marrow) children they treated by combination of rigorous chemotherapy, bone marrow radiotherapy, and stem cell transplants (Rodriguez-Galindo et al. 2003).

Salivary Gland Cancer

There are three major salivary glands on each side of the face. The two parotid glands are the largest and are located over the jaw near the front of the ears. A pair of sublingual glands lies under the floor of the mouth and a pair of submandibular glands are found at the back of the mouth. All six are exocrine glands producing on average 1½ quarts of saliva (watery mix of mucus, salts, and enzymes) that a healthy human generates daily to moisten food for digestion. Saliva also protects teeth from demineralization (tooth decay) by plaque bacteria. There are also a number of much smaller salivary glands decorating the mouth area that are called minor salivary glands.

Salivary gland cancer comprises less than 0.5% of all malignancies worldwide and according to Sun and coworkers (1999) of the National Cancer Institute this disease is associated with atomic bomb survivors and radiotherapy. It is 50% more prevalent in males and not correlated with having AIDS.

The diagnosis of malignant salivary gland tumors is complicated by the fact that it is difficult to distinguish them from the overwhelming majority of tumors that develop and which are benign. Very often a sialogram or ptyalogram, an X-ray of the salivary glands in which a radiopaque dye has been injected in the ducts for increased contrast is required for proper tumor identification.

The parotid gland itself accounts for more than three-fourths of all salivary gland tumors and less than one quarter of these are malignant. Radiotherapy, according to Speight and Barrett (2002) in the U.K. is "a risk factor for malignant change" and so they conclude that the treatment of choice is surgery (parotidectomy) with care given to remove enough of the tumor and surrounding tissue to balance the precarious tradeoff between morbidity and recurrence.

Stage IV tumors of the salivary gland may show invasion of the jaw bone and the base of the skull, and in such cases, neutron beam therapy has been suggested as the treatment of choice with Buchholz and coworkers reporting in 1992 from the University of Washington Medical Center, a most impressive local regional tumor control of 92% after 5 years in 52 men and women.

Because of the limited availability of neutron beam therapy, advanced stage salivary gland cancer patients are more often treated with adjuvant radiotherapy, even though at least one group failed to demonstrate any statistical difference between surgery with and without the post-operative radiotherapy in the 184 men and women so treated.   A 76% 5-year cause specific-survival was common to both treatments (Kirkbride et al. 2001). Adding to an already difficult situation, the National Cancer Institute warns that treating salivary gland tumors with radiotherapy places the patient at increased risk for oropharyngeal, thyroid, and lung cancer (Sun et al. 1999).

Thyroid Cancer

The thyroid gland is a relatively large two-lobed organ that controls growth.   According to the H. Lee Moffitt Cancer Center and Research Institute in Tampa, Florida, cancer of the thyroid gland is relatively rare accounting in 1999 for roughly 1.5% of new cancer cases and less than 0.2% of cancer deaths in the United States. The disease is three times more common in women than men and in the 25 to 65 year age group it has increased in incidence the last decade (McCaffrey 2000).

Thyroid cancers are divided into four types:

Papillary carcinoma represents 80% of all thyroid neoplasms. Follicular carcinoma is the second most common thyroid cancer, accounting for approximately 10% of cases. Medullary thyroid carcinoma represents 5-10% of neoplasms. Anaplastic carcinomas account for 1-2% of cases. (Sharma and Johns 2004)

Except for medullary thyroid carcinoma, exposure to ionizing radiation increases the likelihood of developing thyroid cancer by a factor of up to fifty particularly when subjected to curative radiotherapy of the neck (Jereczek-Fossa et al. 2004). Thyroid cancer can in fact develop as much as 20 years later.   A 1997 study of 284,000 Chernobyl nuclear power plant accident emergency workers determined that each Gy of radiation exposure increased the risk of developing thyroid cancer by more than a factor of five (Ivanov et al. 1997). The 1986 Ukrainian accident has since claimed new victims especially among children who were less than 10-years old at time of exposure (Ivanov et al. 2006).

Both papillary and follicular carcinomas consist of well-differentiated cells that are characteristically slow-growing and consequently highly treatable. Distant metastasis is unlikely and surgery is the most common form of treatment for low-risk patients. A thyroidectomy (surgical removal of all or part of the thyroid gland) is effective if all of the cancerous tissue is removed with 75% 10-year survival rates regularly reported. Adjuvant radioiodine combined with EBRT is used only when there is a high risk of relapse (Brierley and Tsang 1999). A previous year study by Wartofsky of the D.C.'s Washington Hospital Center and by Sherman and Gopal of the Texas M. D. Anderson Cancer Center demonstrated that higher risk thyroid cancer patients are treated with orally administered iodine-131, a beta plus gamma emitter. Notwithstanding this result, a 58-year retrospective study of 727 thyroid cancer patients published in 2004 by Kim and coworkers showed no affect on 20-year overall survival with the implementation of radioactive iodine and only a survival benefit associated with a total thyroidectomy. Around the same time, a British group reported that EBRT doses from 37.5 Gy to 66 Gy are at best controversial in treating thyroid cancer (Ford et al. 2003).

The Memorial Sloan-Kettering Cancer Center in New York City used a 1038 patient retrospective analysis to calculate long-term survival rates of 99%, 87%, and 57% in low-risk, intermediate-risk, and high-risk cancer patients, respectively, concluding that

> surgical treatment offers the best long-term results in low-risk patients, and the role of adjuvant treatment in

this group is questionable.... consideration may be given to external-beam radiation therapy in selected high-risk patients. (Shaha 2004)

Medullary thyroid cancer is the most common type of poorly differentiated thyroid cancer. It affects some 700 people a year in the United States where 44% of the patients are familial and so genetic screening is useful (National Cancer Institute 2006d). The disease has no known treatment (Safioleas et al. 2006).

The rarer anaplastic thyroid cancer is even more deadly and responsible for 40% of all thyroid cancer deaths (Konstantakos and Graham 2006). Treatment is mostly palliative and since the disease is so aggressive, a tracheostomy (surgical opening in the trachea) is frequently required just to promote breathing. Indeed, William H. Rehnquist (1924-2005), the 16th Chief Justice of the U.S. Supreme Court was given a tracheotomy (tracheostomy procedure) a few months before succumbing to this horrible disease.

A Matter of Location

The close proximity of the organs in the head and neck demand extreme treatment care. Table 10.3 shows that radiation has its place here: SRS is aptly applied to the treatment of brain tumors; plaque radiotherapy is overwhelmingly the treatment of choice for cancers of the eye; cancer of the lip is effectively cured with brachytherapy; chemoradiotherapy with IMRT shows promise for nasopharyngeal cancer patients; and neutron beams find use in the treatment of salivary gland cancers. It is important to remember, however, none of these localized treatments deal with the all too common distant metastases that requires a chemotherapeutic remedy.

Table 10.3

Five-year survival rates and preferred treatment
for cancers of the head and neck

Cancer	Survival Rates (%)	Preferred Treatment
Brain	33	Surgery or SRS
Eye	84	Surgery or Plaque Therapy
Hypopharynx	31	Surgery + Radiotherapy (local + regional) Surgery + Chemoradiotherapy (late)
Larynx	84 (local) 50 (regional) 14 (late)	Surgery or Radiotherapy (local + regional) Chemoradiotherapy (late)
Lip	90	Radiotherapy
Nasopharynx	59	Chemoradiotherapy
Oropharynx	36	Surgery + Chemotherapy (local + regional) Chemoradiotherapy (late)
Salivary gland	74	Surgery or Neutron beam therapy
Thyroid	100 (local) 97 (regional) 56 (late)	Surgery
Tongue	56	Surgery (local + regional) Surgery + Radiotherapy (late)

Note: Survival Rates are 5-year relative survival rates (ratio of the proportion of cancer survivors to the proportion of expected survivors) taken from Ries et al. (2006). Preferred Treatment is intended for informational purposes only, is not intended to constitute medical advice, and should not be relied upon in any such regard. Rates and treatment are not stage specific unless otherwise designated as: (local) cancer confined to the organ itself; (regional) cancer extending no further than surrounding tissue; or (late) cancer has metastasized to distant organs.

Digestive System Cancers

The digestive system allows for the breakdown of foods into the chemicals that fuel the body. This system of organs encompasses a contiguous and highly convoluted tubular path that begins with the mouth and ends with the anus and includes the esophagus, stomach, and small and large intestine in between. Other organs, such as the salivary glands, liver, gallbladder, and pancreas, are also an integral part of the digestive system, although no foods actually pass through any of these organs.

Digestive system cancers are, perhaps because of all the substances including the carcinogens and toxins that pass through them, collectively the most frequently occurring cancers in the world (table 11.1). Colorectal (colon and rectum) and stomach cancer are after lung and breast cancer the third and fourth most commonly diagnosed cancers worldwide. Colorectal cancer is associated with obesity, lack of physical activity, low consumption of fruit and vegetables (Danaei et al. 2005) and with the prolonged long-term consumption of red and

Table 11.1

Worldwide incidence of digestive system cancers

Cancer	Incidence (cases per year)
Colorectal	1,033,000
Stomach	934,000
Liver	626,000
Esophagus	462,000
Pancreas	232,000

Source: Mackay et al. (2006).

processed meat (cured, dried, pickled, salted, smoked, etc.) according to Chao and coworkers (2005). Reacting to people's eating habits, the American Cancer Society's chief of epidemiology warns that

> for people who reported high consumption of red meat and processed meat ... that is long-term high consumption, we found about a 50 percent higher risk of colon cancer. (American Cancer Society 2005b)

Table 11.2 shows the incidence of colorectal cancer is roughly the same in all four industrialized countries. Stomach cancer, on the other hand, is five to eight times more prevalent in Japan. In the United States, Asian-Americans and Pacific Islanders have the highest incidence of this disease suggesting that these people are racially and/or culturally predisposed to stomach cancer (U.S. Department of Health and Human Services 2005).

Stomach cancer is associated with smoking and diets lacking in fruits and vegetables (Danaei et al. 2005). It is also a disease that is casually linked to infection from *Helicobacter pylori* (*H pylori*), an oncogenic bacteria, that is present in most people's stomachs (Ando et al. 2006; Crew and Neugut 2006). Nothing is ever simple in life with Ye and coworkers (2004) reporting that *H pylori* is reduces the risk of cancer of the esophagus.

Table 11.2

New cases of cancer of the digestive system
diagnosed annually per 100,000 population

Cancer	U.S.	Canada	Japan	U.K.
Anus	1.6	-	-	-
Bowel	-	60.4	-	43.8
Colon	35.8	-	35.1	-
Esophagus	4.9	4.5	8.9	9.5
Gallbladder	2.9	-	(13.4)	-
Liver	6.2	-	21.8	3.4
Pancreas	11.3	10.6	10.4	8.6
Rectum	14.1	-	19.0	-
Small intestine	2.1	-	-	-
Stomach	7.5	8.5	60.9	11.2

Source: Jemal et al. (2006); Canadian Cancer Society (2006);
National Cancer Center (2005); Cancer Research UK (2002);
U.S. Central Intelligence Agency (2006).
Note: Bowel statistics for Canada include the colon and rectum, and
for the U.K. include the anus, colon, rectum, and small intestine.
Rates are age-adjusted and (crude).

Liver cancer, the fifth most common cancer in the world, is linked to both smoking and drinking. It is also caused by the hepatitis B virus (HBV) and the hepatitis C virus (HCV)—two oncogenic agents transmitted by the blood (Danaei et al. 2005). Since 1982, HBV has been prevented by vaccine at birth in the United States and elsewhere. In Japan, where liver cancer is far more prevalent than in the United States and the U.K., Yoshizawa (2002) attributed liver cancer to HCV, a result of the widespread use of intravenous methamphetamine (speed) at the end of World War II.

Liver cancer is also linked to exposure to vinyl chloride, a sweet-smelling, colorless gas that is integral to the plastics industry (Boffetta et al. 2003); Bosetti et al. 2003). The gas is polymerized to make polyvinyl chloride (PVC) and is listed in the United States as a "known carcinogen" by the Environmental Protection Agency (2000) and as a "potential occupational carcinogen" by the National Institute for Occupational Safety and Health (2005b). In addition, there is a further relationship between HBV infection and liver cancer in men exposed to vinyl chloride fumes according to Wong and coworkers (2003) in Taiwan where the majority of vinyl chloride workers have a history of HBV infection.

Malignancies of the digestive system are among the most lethal cancers in the world, killing 1.56 times more men than women, the overwhelming majority of which are 45-years and older. The most deadly cancers of the digestive system—stomach, liver, and colorectal—each kill more people annually than breast cancer, a disease that causes the death of 502,000 men and women per year.

Stomach cancer, the second most deadly cancer, kills 912,000 people per year and 1.61 more men than women. Liver cancer, the third deadliest cancer in the world and the second deadliest digestive system cancer, kills 2.26 times more men then women. Colorectal cancer, the world's fourth deadliest, kills just about the same number of men and women as does pancreatic cancer, a disease with a mortality that is comparable to cancers of the cervix and prostate (World Health Organization 2005a).

Table 11.3

Worldwide deaths from digestive system cancers

Cancer	Mortality (deaths per year)	
	Male	Female
Stomach	563,000	349,000
Liver	459,000	203,000
Colorectal	342,000	314,000
Esophagus	306,000	175,000
Pancreas	128,000	114,000

Source: World Health Organization 2005a.

Canada has the highest colorectal cancer mortality (table 11.4). In Japan and the U.K., where colorectal cancer mortality is the same as in the United States, cancer of the colon is twice as deadly as cancer of the rectum. Stomach cancer and liver cancer are several times more deadly in Japan than in the United States, Canada, and the U.K. The mortality rates for cancer of the esophagus and the pancreas are comparable in all four countries. The higher mortality rate for cancer of the gallbladder in Japan

Table 11.4

Yearly deaths from cancer of the digestive system per 100,000 population

Cancer	U.S.	Canada	Japan	U.K.
Colorectal	18.5	25.7	18.3	18.6
Esophagus	4.6	5.0	5.9	8.7
Gallbladder	1.1	-	(5.1)	-
Liver	5.4	-	17.0	3.2
Pancreas	10.8	10.3	9.9	8.5
Stomach	3.8	5.6	24.1	6.9

Source: Jemal et al. (2006); Canadian Cancer Society (2006); National Cancer Center (2005); Cancer Research UK (2002); U.S. Central Intelligence Agency (2006).
Note: Rates are age-adjusted and (crude).

compared to the United States is reflective of the higher incidence in Japan (table 11.2).

Anal Cancer

Anal cancer is rare and when it does occur it usually develops in the outer part of the anus in males and the anal canal in females. The anus is the last 1 inch or so end of the large intestine after the rectum. Essentially a ring like muscle, it serves to discharge fecal material.

Cancer of the anus is more common in women than in men and is considered highly curable in both sexes as long as it has not spread to distant organs. In stage I, the cancer is less than 1 inch in diameter, in stage II it is larger than 1 inch in diameter, and in stage III it is any size and has advanced to nearby lymph nodes.

Risk factors that contribute to this disease include smoking, being over 50 years of age, engaging in anal intercourse, and contracting the HPV. Homosexual males are more than thirty times as likely to develop anal cancer as heterosexual males. Female homosexuals show no such correlation.

Chemoradiotherapy is the treatment of choice. A group in Germany achieved 71% 5-year overall survival with 45 Gy dose EBRT administered in fractions of 2 Gy and less (Graf et al. 2003). To increase local tumor control EBRT and iridium-192 brachytherapy are often combined with chemotherapy. In this way, Vordermark and coworkers (2001) achieved 84% 5-year overall survival in 20 patients, Deniaud-Alexandre and coworkers (2003) reported 74% 10-year disease-free survival rates in 305 patients, and Dubois, Azria, and Ychou (2003) claimed a 5-year overall survival of 91% in 70 patients. Most of the people treated had stage II cancers, and in all cases the side effects of this combined treatment therapy included the risk of colostomy (surgically created opening to the large intestine for collecting waste).

Biliary Tract Cancer

The gallbladder is a non-essential organ found in humans, dogs and cats, but not in horses and rats. It lies on the right side of the body beneath the liver where it stores bile—a green fluid used in the digestion and absorption of fats. Adults produce 1 pint or so of bile a day. Bile aids in the dissolution and elimination of cholesterol (steroid precursor produced and consumed by the body), which if precipitates, form what are commonly called gallstones. The gallbladder is connected to the liver and the small intestine by a series of tubes called the bile duct.

Cancer of the gallbladder accounts for about two-thirds of biliary tract cancers and is more common in females and those who have a history of gallstones (Randi, Franceschi, La Vecchia 2006). Because its symptoms—stomach pains, headaches, and fever—are similar to many other illnesses, it is rarely detected early enough to be curative.

If the tumor is stage I or II, and if it is confined to the muscle layer, then surgery is 100% curable and a cholecystectomy, the complete removal of the gallbladder is typical. If however the cancer has spread to a blood vessel in the liver or to a nearby organ, survival is reduced to less than 5 years (Behari et al. 2003).

Unfortunately most gallbladder cancers cannot be treated by surgery alone and thus, Leone and coworkers (2002) in Italy relied on liver resection in addition to a cholecystectomy to achieve 20% 5-year survival rates for stage III but no success for stage IV. Similarly, Ito and coworkers (2004) of the Harvard Medical School achieved 13% 5-year survival in 48 men and women treated over a 20-year period. A group in Mexico compared surgery to resection combined with adjuvant EBRT in a 45 patient retrospective study and found that surgery alone favors the patient; 100% 5-year survival versus 39% to 62% depending on the cancer stage (Mondragon-Sanchez et al. 2003).

Bile duct cancer, also called cholangiocarcinoma is rare outside of Asia. The most common form of biliary cancer is extrahepatic, which is curable by surgery in only 10% of all cases. The Mayo Clinic in Rochester, Minnesota points out that this cancer is especially difficult to diagnose and that early detection is key to survival as the disease readily metastasizes to the liver and even then, liver transplantation coupled with preoperative chemoradiotherapy is deemed necessary (Gores 2000).

A University of Southern California retrospective study showed that when surgery is possible, the 5-year survival rate in 38 men and 39 women is as high as 55% (Blom and Schwartz 2001). Others in the United States share a similar point of view concluding that 44% 5-year survival is reasonable (Johnson et al. 2001).

A recent South Korean retrospective study by Kim and coworkers (2002) concluded that chemoradiotherapy with >40 Gy EBRT after surgery does not improve overall survival rates when used adjuvantly. The Mayo Clinic points out that it is long known that such adjuvant therapy increases complications from gastric bleeding and inflammation of the bile duct while failing to treat distant metastasis and local tumor recurrence (Foo et al. (1997).

In the incurable cases, Crane et al. of the Texas M. D. Anderson Cancer Center and Gonzalez Gonzalez et al. in the Netherlands have used a combined modality treatment that included EBRT, chemotherapy, and iridium-192 brachytherapy boosts to give, in some cases, a 10-month survival rate. Cameron and coworkers (1990) of the Baltimore John Hopkins Hospital and van Berkel and coworkers (2004) in the Netherlands add that palliative therapies often include stenting the biliary vessel wall.

Colon Cancer

Colon cancer specifies malignancies that originate in the first 5 feet or so of the large intestine (place where moisture is extracted from the digested residue following the small intestine). Defecation—the passage of fecal waste or stool—is a partly voluntary and partly involuntary act that occurs as often as two or three times a day and as infrequently as every other day depending on the person and the diet. There is no relationship between the frequency of defecating and the incidence of these cancers.

The colon is muscular multilayered organ. When cancer develops here it is considered treatable with survival depending on tumor size and staging: stage 0 cancer also called carcinoma *in situ* or intramucosal carcinoma has not grown beyond the inner layer of the colon; stage I (sometimes referred to as Duke's A colon cancer) extends into the middle layers of the colon; stage II (Duke's B colon cancer) has penetrated beyond the middle layers of the colon and may have even spread to another organ; stage III (Duke's C colon cancer) has spread to three or more lymph nodes; and stage IV (Duke's D colon cancer) involves nearby lymph nodes and one or more other organs.

The University of Pennsylvania School of Medicine states that early stage colon cancer can be cured with surgery (El-Deiry 2006). The Yale University School of Medicine further adds that at the time of diagnosis, 28% of all colon cancer patients are stage II, and 37% are stage III, both of which can be treated by surgery with patients expecting to be cured 60% to 80% of the time and 30% to 60% of the time respectively (Saif 2006). Even stage IV colon cancer patients are said to benefit from surgical resection, a treatment that can improve 1-year survival from 12% without surgery to 45% with surgery (Cook, Single, and McCahill 2005). Moreover, in some cases, where only the cancerous portion of the colon is removed, the remaining healthy parts may be surgically reconnected; a procedure that is called intestinal anastomosis.

Irrespective of all this, 40% to 50% of those who undergo surgery will suffer relapse primarily due to previously undetected metastatic tumors or metastasis to the liver. If the liver is surgically removed, a 26% to 49% 5-year survival rate can be realized. In some cases where liver resection is not initially feasible, chemotherapy can be implemented to allow for liver resection to take place achieving similar 5-year survival rates (Biasco, et al. 2006). In the most advanced cases, of colon cancer surgery is also used palliatively (El-Deiry 2006).

Esophageal Cancer

The esophagus begins where the hypopharynx ends. Cancer of the esophagus—a 10-inch long tube that connects the throat to the stomach is often called esophageal cancer (or oesophageal in Commonwealth English). Surgery is most commonly prescribed if the cancer has not spread, but by the time most esophageal tumors are detected, the cancer has metastasized and surgery is no longer curative:

> Neither surgery nor radiation therapy reliably provides long-term control for patients, even with apparently localized disease.... Radiotherapy can thus not be recommended as a single modality treatment or as the only adjuvant therapy with surgery in a curative approach. Radiotherapy has been of little value in converting unresectable cancers into respectable ones. (Albertsson 2002)

In 2003, Makary and coworkers of the Georgetown University Hospital in Washington D.C. reported 38% 5-year survival rates in 40 patients using neoadjuvant chemoradiotherapy before surgery, an improvement over surgery alone even with larger tumors. At the same time a John Hopkins group in neighboring Baltimore achieved 40% 5-year survival in 92 people noting no difference in survival or response between those with adenocarcinoma or squamous cell carcinoma (Kleinberg et al. 2003). A second chemoradiotherapy study of 236 patients at the Memorial Sloan-Kettering Cancer Center in New York City showed 2-year survival rates of 31% to 40% and no difference with high (64.8 Gy) versus low (50.4 Gy) dose radiation except that 11 high dose patients died (Minsky et al. 2002).

Lastly, Homs and coworkers (2006) in the Netherlands report palliative benefits of using 12 Gy brachytherapy to deal with the dysphagia (difficulty swallowing) that so often accompanies this cancer.

Gastrointestinal Carcinoids

Carcinoids are small benign or malignant tumors originating anywhere in the gastrointestinal (GI) tract that secrete serotonin—a brain chemical associated with sleep and mood. All GI carcinoids, except for those found in the rectum, produce endocrine substances.

GI carcinoid tumors develop from cells that help regulate digestive juices and the muscle movement of food products through the intestines. They account for less than 2% of all digestive system cancers in the United States. Carcinoids are slow growing and are frequently found in the appendix (pouch-like organ of unknown function located on the right side of the body adjacent the colon). There is no acceptable staging for these malignancies.

A monumental 1950 to 1999 analysis of 13,715 people with this disease by Modlin and coworkers of the Yale University School of Medicine published in 2003 showed the following: two-thirds of all carcinoids show up in the GI tract, 42% in the small intestine, 27% in the rectum, and 9% in the stomach; females account for 55% of all carcinoid tumor patients with 61 years the average age of diagnosis; African American males have, at 4.5 per 100,000 population (age-adjusted), the highest incidence of any group; and distant metastases is evident at time of diagnosis in 13% of all patients leading to a 67% 5-year overall survival rate (1992-1999) for all stages and sites.

If GI carcinoids are found there is a 46% chance that additional localized tumors are present (Gerstle, Kauffman Jr., and Koltun 1995). Even then, a person can expect to live at least 2 years after diagnosis due to the slow tumor growth. For both sexes, workers in Sweden claim that the 5-year and 15-year overall survival is approximately 60% and 25% respectively, for tumors surgically removed from the small intestine (Zar et al. 2004).

The M. D. Anderson Cancer Center in Houston, Texas reports that malignant carcinoids that have metastasized to other sites are incurable due to the high toxicity and poor efficacy of chemotherapy (Schnirer, Yao, and Ajani 2003). Addressing this problem, the Yale University School of Medicine demonstrated that intravenously administered indium-111 (2.83 day half-life emitting 0.171 and 0.245 MeV gamma rays and 23 keV X-rays) tagged somatostatin (growth inhibiting hormone), RIT, and interferon (host-specific antiviral agent), were somewhat effective in treating metastatic disease resulting in a 33% 5-year overall survival rate (Modlin et al. 2005).

Liver Cancer

The liver is the largest internal organ in the body. It filters impurities and toxins in the blood and aids in digestion. Occupying most of the right side of the abdomen and weighing some 3 pounds, this reddish-brown organ is the main source for converting excess carbohydrates and proteins into fat that is stored elsewhere. The liver is capable of regenerating itself when injured or diseased.

Hepatocellular carcinomas begin in adult liver cells. For certain localized tumors, according to Fong's group (1999) at the Memorial Sloan-Kettering Cancer Center in the United States and Chang and coworkers (2004) in Taiwan, surgery is the best treatment offering 50% 5-year survival rates in people without cirrhosis (irreversible scarring of liver tissue associated with alcoholism and hepatitis). A French group adds that since tumor recurrence is likely, adjuvant radiotherapy with iodine-131 injected directly into the bloodstream after surgery is beneficial (Boucher et al. 2003). Iodine-131's relatively short 8-day half-life causes all of its radiation to be dissipated within 3 months.

In males and females whose localized tumors are not resectable, prognosis is poor and other novel forms of treatment such as cryosurgery and radioablation are utilized, but mostly for palliation (Nordlinger and Rougier 2002).

The University of Michigan Medical Center reported treating 22 hepatobiliary patients (11 hepatocellular carcinoma and 11 cholangiocarcinoma) with 48 Gy or 66 Gy EBRT to achieve a 20% 4-year overall survival rate (Robertson et al. 1997). Several years later, Cheng and coworkers (2002) in Taiwan reported that because of the concern for radiation-induced liver disease, EBRT is not commonly used. Recognizing the need for a more conformal radiation source, a German group concluded that SRS is preferable:

> Stereotactic single-dose radiation therapy is a feasible method for the treatment of singular inoperable liver metastases with the potential of high local tumor control rate and low morbidity. (Herfarth et al. 2001)

Alternatively confining the radiation to the cancerous tissue with brachytherapy, the Ohio State University used 160 Gy iodine-125 permanent seed implants to treat 64 unresectable and metastatic liver cancer patients and achieved 73%, 23%, and 5% 1-year, 3-year, and 5-year overall survival rates, respectively (Nag et al. 2006).

Pancreatic Cancer

The pancreas is a nominally 6-inch long pear shaped organ that sits on the left side of the body behind the stomach and in front of the spine. It is a two-part gland; the exocrine part neutralizes stomach acid and produces enzymes that digest proteins and breakdown starches—the carbohydrates found in potatoes, corn, wheat, and the like; the endocrine part, often called the islets of Langerhans, releases insulin, a hormone that regulates blood sugar.

The pancreas is a most essential organ in that without it we would starve in spite of eating healthy. Like the kidney, it can be transplanted, but transplants are not used to remedy pancreatic cancer because pancreatic cancer cells tend to break away and show up elsewhere.

Certain people are genetically predisposed to this disease and in the United States 5% to 10% of all cases are familial with more than 600 families having more than one close relative (parent, child, or sibling) diagnosed with pancreatic cancer (Johns Hopkins Pancreas Cancer Web 2005).

Four months is the median survival for exocrine pancreatic cancer, the most common form, according to the Washington University School of Medicine in Missouri, almost all of which are adenocarcinomas (Fesinmeyer et al. 2005). If the disease is localized and resectable, and this is the case 20% of the time, even then the prognosis is not good. The California Cancer Registry studied 10,612 people with exocrine pancreatic cancer noting 3.5 months and 13.3 months median survival for unresected and resected patients respectively (Cress et al. 2006). The New York City Memorial Sloan-Kettering Cancer Center reported 10% 5-year survival after surgery in people treated between 1983 and 1989, a result that they emphasize is not curative.

The most common pancreatic surgery is known as the Whipple procedure (pancreaticoduodenectomy). It is a nominal 4 to 7 hour long surgical operation in which the head of the pancreas (wide part adjacent the beginning of the small intestine), the gallbladder, the bile duct, and a portion of the stomach and small intestine, are removed (Conlon, Klimstra, and Brennan 1996):

> Pancreatic cancer is a devastating disease characterized by a dismal prognosis with most patients dying within six months after diagnosis. Surgery is an option in less than one in five of these patients, and even with tumor resection the majority of patients succumb to the disease. Other effective treatment options are not available. (Hennig, Ding, and Adrian 2004)

Sixteen members of the European Study Group for Pancreatic Cancer reported in 2004 a study of 289 resectable pancreatic cancer patients with a median follow-up of 47 months listing 237 deaths and concluding that chemotherapy alone was marginally beneficial, whereas chemoradiotherapy had a deleterious effect on survival:

> One can only conclude that after nearly ten years of work and nearly 600 patients studied, that post-operative radiotherapy is positively harmful after pancreatic resection for cancer. [The European Study Group for Pancreatic Cancer] have simply confirmed the negative and/or inconclusive results of the impact of adjuvant chemotherapy seen in all the previous trials. (Poston 2004)

If the tumor is not surgically removable and the cancer has neither metastasized nor spread to the lymph nodes, Moertel and 28 other members of the international Gastrointestinal Tumor Study Group (1981) reported that chemoradiotherapy lead to a 1-year survival improvement over radiotherapy alone—an impressive 40% versus 10% in the 194 people so treated. Unfortunately, according to the Thomas Jefferson University Hospital, in Philadelphia, Pennsylvania, median survival rates are still not much greater than 14 months when a chemotherapy, pre-operative EBRT regime was used to treat 88 patients between 1974 and 1981, noting however that the addition of iodine-125 brachytherapy increased survival in 30% to 18 months (Whittington et al. (1984).

Twenty years later, pancreatic cancer remains no less formidable. This is nowhere better illustrated than in a German study reporting 1-year and 2-year survival of 53% and 18% respectively in 17 patients neoadjuvantly treated with hypofractionated radiotherapy and chemotherapy (Zimmerman et al. 2004). One year later Micke and coworkers (2005) also in Germany reported that a chemotherapy regiment combined with hyperfractionated 44.8 Gy radiotherapy gave 55% 1-year survival, and 24% 2-year survival; median survival was 13.8 months.

Endocrine pancreatic cancer is a different beast altogether—it is curable. In the summer of 2004, Steve Jobs, the cofounder of Apple Computer was diagnosed with islet cell neuroendocrine carcinoma, Jobs' physician noting that

> he will not need radiation or chemotherapy.... If you remove all of the tumor, there is a high probability the patient is cured. (Stanford University Medical Center 2004)

Cancer of the Rectum

Rectal cancer refers to malignant tumors located in the rectum, the last 6 inches of the large intestine where feces are stored prior to defecation. Cancer of the rectum is staged and for the most part treated in the same manner as colon cancer. Rectal cancers are surgically cured in approximately 45% of all cases with adjuvant radiotherapy used when the disease is localized.

A Swedish group of surgeons reported that 557 people with rectal cancer who had received pre-operative radiotherapy obtained 46% 8-year overall survival rates compared to 39% who did not receive the radiation benefit. Within 6 months of surgery, 5% of the patients treated with radiotherapy died of non-cancerous causes, mainly of cardiovascular disease (Martling et al. 2001). At the same time, a group from the Netherlands reported local tumor control in 1805 patients treated with preoperative radiotherapy, however noting no improvement in overall survival (Kapiteijn et al. 2001).

In 1991, Krook and coworkers of the Duluth Community Clinical Oncology Program in Minnesota reported that 204 rectal carcinoma patients in which the disease had spread beyond the rectum and treated with adjuvant chemoradiotherapy showed 36% fewer cancer-related deaths and 29% less deaths overall, but not without chemoradiotherapy side effects that included nausea, vomiting, and diarrhea (all characteristic symptoms of radiation enteritis), a reduced white blood cell count, and bowel obstruction that required additional surgery in 14 patients.

Three years later, the Mayo Clinic, also in Minnesota, stated that

> adjuvant postoperative chemoradiotherapy for rectal carcinoma has a major long-term detrimental effect on bowel function (Kollmorgen et al. 1994)

on the basis of a retrospective study of 100 people 2 to 5 years post-treatment. The National Surgical Adjuvant Breast and Bowel Project added that monitoring stage II (outside the rectum without nodal involvement) and stage III (nodal involvement without distant metastasis) cancer patients in the United States for up to 93 months following chemotherapy with and without radiotherapy showed no beneficial disease-free or overall survival rates (Wolmark et al. 2000).

Cancer of the Small Intestine

The small intestine or bowel as it is sometimes referred is the nominal 22 feet of the digestive tract connecting the stomach to the colon. It is the main place of digestion accounting for 90% of the body's digestive absorptive surface area. The first 10 inches or so of the small intestine and also its widest part is called the duodenum. More than just a conduit, the duodenum is interestingly enough another endocrine gland.

In the United States, cancer of the small intestine is almost twice as common in blacks as it is in whites (Stanford University's Haselkorn, Whittemore, and Lilienfeld 2005). Most cancers of the small intestine are adenocarcinomas occurring in the duodenum. The Columbia University College of Physicians and Surgeons lists risk factors as being male, smoking cigarettes, drinking alcohol, and having peptic ulcers (Neugut et al. 1998).

New York's Mount Sinai Medical Center notes that adenocarcinomas of the small intestine are markedly more difficult to deal with than malignant carcinoid tumors in the same organ having median survival of 13 months and 36 months respectively. Mount Sinai further reports that cure rates are entirely dependent on how fully resectable the tumor is and that adjuvant chemotherapy or radiotherapy does not affect survival, which after the all too common tumor recurrence is very poor (Cunningham et al. 1997).

Recently, the M. D. Anderson Cancer Center evaluated 217 patients and found 4% at stage I, 20% at stage II, 39%

at stage III, and 35% at stage IV with the liver being the most common metastatic site. Surgery was possible for 67% of the patients with a 26% 5-year overall survival result (Dabaja et al. 2004).

Stomach Cancer

The stomach is a muscular saclike organ on the left side of the abdomen where digestion begins in earnest. It is expandable having a volume that varies from as little as 0.01 liter to more than 1 to 2 liters between meals.

Cancer of the stomach, often called gastric cancer, has changed over the last 20 years in the United States with tumors that were primarily located near the connection to the intestines (distal end) now more commonly located near the connection to the esophagus (proximal end). The University of Utah and Tulane University collaboratively reported that in all cases of stomach cancer a 23% 5-year overall survival is realizable (Hazard, O'Connor, and Scaife 2006). The death rate from recurrent stomach cancer is roughly 75% according to the Saint Vincent's Comprehensive Cancer Center in New York City (MacDonald 2003).

Surgery is the overwhelming treatment of choice especially for those patients with stage I and II gastric tumors in which the cancer is localized and does not extend beyond the stomach. A group in Spain warns that in general, people with stomach cancer have a low overall survival rate because even in these early stages the disease has inevitably migrated to other organs and so alternate therapies are required (Grau et al. 2003).

Locally advanced gastric cancer is typically treated with neoadjuvant chemotherapy and according to a German clinic, 76% of the tumors in 49 patients were successfully resected after chemotherapy to achieve a median survival of 32 months (Ott et al. 2003).

A recent study of 556 resected gastric cancer patients showed overall survival going from 27 months with surgery alone to 36 months for surgery combined with chemoradiotherapy. And in spite of side effects requiring 41% of the patients to undergo minor surgical intervention or hospital admission and 32% major surgical intervention and a long hospital stay, this treatment regime has become the standard of care (MacDonald et al. 2001). The Dana-Farber Cancer Institute in Boston criticized the MacDonald study noting that

> much of the benefit of chemoradiation in this trial appears to relate to improved local control rather than prevention of distant disease

further emphasizing that only 65% of the patients completed the treatment (Meyerhardt and Fuchs 2003). A group in Japan also criticized the Macdonald group study:

> Since most of the patients treated with potentially curative surgery still have dismal prognosis in the West, investigators there do not hesitate to introduce toxic regimens.... Chemoradiation has not been seriously explored in Japan where investigators believe that local control can be achieved through extended [surgery]. (Kodera et al. 2006)

A 22-year retrospective analysis of 314 people with stomach cancer treated with surgery plus chemoradiotherapy demonstrated a 5-year actuarial survival rate of 60%. Side effects included 25% of the patients experiencing blood clotting, 22% having a decrease in white blood cell count, and 12% vomiting without need for an extended hospital stay; adding that an advantage of chemotherapy without radiotherapy is that patients accepted the treatment better (Grau et al. 2003).

For the 60% of the people with gastric cancer, the tumors are not confined to the stomach and are thus unresectable. Here, chemoradiotherapy appears to give a survival benefit, ·

> however, the use of combined-modality therapy in unresectable gastric cancer is tempered by the fact that relatively few of these patients will be long-term survivors. (Hazard, O'Connor, and Scaife 2006)

Less than 3% of the people who develop stomach cancer are genetically predisposed to develop hereditary diffuse gastric cancer, a poorly differentiated adenocarcinoma (Fitzgerald and Caldas 2004):

> The average age of onset of hereditary diffuse gastric cancer is 38 years, with a range of 14-69 years.... The estimated cumulative risk of gastric cancer by age 80 years is 67% for men and 83% for women. Women also have a 39% risk for lobular breast cancer. (Kaurah and Huntsman 2004)

Tough to Swallow

The prognosis for cancers of the digestive system is overall unsettling (table 11.5). Statistically, cancers of the liver and the stomach are just as deadly today as they were more than 2 decades ago and the 5-year survival rates of all stages of almost all cancers of the biliary tract, esophagus, gallbladder, and pancreas are equally depressing.

A few digestive system cancers, notably those of the lower GI tract, are treatable especially if discovered early. Brachytherapy and EBRT, for example, are equally effective in the chemoradiotherapeutic treatment of anal cancer and colorectal cancers and carcinoid tumors are often surgically removed with great success.

Table 11.5

Five-year survival rates and preferred treatment
for cancers of the digestive system

Cancer	Survival Rates (%)	Preferred Treatment
Anus	66	Chemoradiotherapy
Biliary duct	6	Surgery (local + regional) Surgery + Chemoradiotherapy (late)
Colon	90 (local) 68 (regional) 10 (late)	Surgery (local + regional) Surgery + Chemotherapy (late)
Esophagus	34 (local) 17 (regional) 3 (late)	Surgery (local + regional) Chemoradiotherapy (late)
Gallbladder	15	Surgery
GI carcinoid	67	Surgery (local + regional) RIT (late)
Liver	22 (local) 7 (regional) 3 (late)	Surgery (local + regional) Brachytherapy (late)
Pancreas	20 (local) 8 (regional) 2 (late)	Surgery (local + regional) Chemoradiotherapy (late)
Rectum	90 (local) 68 (regional) 10 (late)	Surgery
Small intestine	56	Surgery
Stomach	62 local) 22 (regional) 3 (late)	Surgery (local + regional) Surgery + Chemoradiotherapy (late)

Note: Survival Rates are 5-year relative survival rates (ratio of the proportion of cancer survivors to the proportion of expected survivors) taken from Ries et al. (2006); Modlin, Lye, and Kidd (2003). Preferred Treatment is intended for informational purposes only, is not intended to constitute medical advice, and

Table 11.5 (continued)

should not be relied upon in any such regard. Rates and treatment are not stage specific unless otherwise designated as: (local) cancer confined to the organ itself; (regional) cancer extending no further than surrounding tissue; or (late) cancer has metastasized to distant organs.

Surviving cancer is very often a matter of knowledge. Knowing that their family had a bad gene, 11 cousins opted to have their stomachs removed rather than risk a 70% chance of developing hereditary diffuse gastric cancer. All six of the cousins who had their stomachs surgically resected at the Stanford University Medical Center, Stanford, California, were diagnosed with early tumors that were discovered in their stomachs only after they had been removed (Daily News Central 2006). For these people, quality of life is living without a stomach.

Benign Tumors and Other Maladies

A benign tumor is usually only a serious health problem when it begins to occupy valuable space in the body and nowhere is that space more precious than inside the human skull. The skull is entirely bone and very much alive growing the first 7 years or so of its life, whereupon it is then forever sealed. A hardened vault composed of 30 different bones, the skull houses and protects the brain and primary sensory organs—eyes, ears, nose, and the tongue. The brain grows from less than 1 pound at birth to nearly 3 pounds at 15 years at which point the brain changes little in size.

With the volume of the skull permanently fixed, radiation is aptly applied to the treatment of almost any intracranial growth that threatens to compete with healthy brain tissue for the limited space available. And unlike surgery which requires a craniotomy (removal of a portion of the bone and its replacement following the procedure) radiotherapy does not break the integrity of the skull, as the beam of ionizing radiation literally penetrates through the skull without causing it any physical harm.

Several types of benign tumors and other maladies are of interest to radiotherapy. In brief, anything that can be "treated" with a surgeon's scalpel can be treated with a radiologist's beam.

Acoustic Neurinoma

Acoustic neuromas are a slow growing mass of tissue that develop from nerve cells between the ear and the brain in mostly 30 to 60 year old women and which if left untreated can ultimately be life threatening. Why these tumors develop is unknown, but approximately 2.5% of the general U.S. population has been found post-mortem to have them and some without ever experiencing symptoms that include hearing loss, ringing in the ears (tinnitus), dizziness (vertigo), difficulty in balance, and facial paralysis (Levine 1999). If hearing loss is reported, it is never regained even with treatment.

SRS is useful in retarding acoustic neurinoma growth. One retrospective study demonstrated that at least in the Netherlands, radiosurgery is a more cost effective treatment than the more conventional microsurgery even while acknowledging that radiation rarely destroys these benign tumors altogether (van Roijen et al. 1997):

> Approximately 20% of tumors continue to grow after radiosurgery or at some time in the future. A tumor which has been irradiated and grows may be more difficult to remove than an un-radiated tumor.... In the long term radiosurgery is more expensive than microsurgery because it requires follow-up. (Levine 1999)

According to a report from Melbourne, Australia, surgery is very effective in treating these small tumors while radiotherapy seems to be best at inhibiting tumor growth (Meyer et al. 2006). However, in at least one case, 30 Gy Gamma Knife surgery transformed a benign acoustic neuroma into a malignant tumor where the patient died 6.5 years after treatment (Kenchiro et al. 2001).

Bone Pain

Aches and pains in the bone brought on by metastasis, leukemia, multiple myeloma, osteoporosis (a degenerative disease characterized by demineralization of the bone and which affects upwards of 10 million people in the United States alone) and other trauma such as a fracture, are collectively referred to as bone pain. Bone pain that results from metastasis is the most common cause of pain in cancer patients according to the City of Hope National Medical Center (Slatkin 2006). Radiotherapy is used to treat bone pain and provide an 80% overall response (Hoskin 2003). A review of clinical trials concludes that with EBRT

> almost two thirds of patients will experience improvement in their pain, with complete and long-lasting pain relief in about half of the patients. (Vakeat and Boterberg 2004)

A group in Australia reported success in treating bone pain with EBRT using 8 Gy (single-dose) or 20 Gy in 5 dose fractions achieving an impressive complete response (no sensation of pain) in 27% of those treated (Roos et al. 2005). Injecting strontium-89 (1.46 MeV beta emitter with a 50.5-day half-life) and samarium-153 (combination 825 keV beta and 103 keV gamma emitter with a 46.7-hour half-life) radioisotopes into the bloodstream provided pain relief to greater than 60% of 8051 people so treated (Falkmer et al. 2003).

Alternatively and with great success, orally administered or infused bisphosphonate (harmless organic phosphorus salts) drugs are widely being administered to treat bone pain (Falkmer et al. 2003; Coleman 2004; Vakeat and Boterberg 2004).

Craniopharyngioma

A craniopharyngioma is a benign tumor that also develops within the skull near the pituitary gland. It accounts for roughly 5% of all primary brain tumors and as much as 10% of all pediatric brain tumors. Craniopharyngiomas are most commonly found in children 5 to 14 years of age and in adults older than 65 years having no known environmental risk factors or genetic predisposition (Haupt et al. 2006).

Craniopharyngiomas are most frequently removed by surgery, even though tumor recurrence is a well known problem. Because of a high morbidity associated with resecting recurring tumors, SRS is beneficial in treating such tumors achieving 5-year recurrence free survival rates as high as 80% (Habrand et al. 1999; Baraua et al. 2003).

Cushing Disease

Cushing disease or Cushing's syndrome primarily results from a benign tumor in the brain's pituitary gland. It is a rare disease, affecting 10 to 15 in 1,000,000 people, primarily age 20 to 50 years, and women five times more so than men (National Institute of Diabetes and Digestive and Kidney Diseases 2002). Also called hypercortisolism, this disease is the result of the pituitary gland sending the wrong signal to the adrenal gland, which then overproduces cortisol—the so-called flight-or-fight hormone. This overproduction typically manifests itself as upper body obesity with thinning arms and legs and thin, fragile skin. Women tend to grow hair on their face and chest and men tend to have decreased fertility and sexual drive.

Surgical removal of the pituitary gland (adenomectomy) is reported to cure 91% of 34 people treated according to a 10-year review of Sweden's Karolinksa Hospital procedures (Hoybye et al. 2004). Alternatively, the Texas M. D. Anderson Cancer Center recently claimed that SRS obtained 90% remission (reduction in tumor volume) in Cushing disease patients. Accompanying treatment were few incidences of radiation-induced complications such as vision loss and secondary cancers causing this institute to conclude that cure rates with radiotherapy were equal to surgery (Hentschel and McCutcheon 2004).

Epilepsy

In the U.K., the National Society for Epilepsy claims that 40 million people worldwide have epilepsy, a condition that is defined as having had two or more epileptic seizures. An estimated 2½ million Americans have had or will have an epileptic seizure (a sometimes violent and always uncontrollable contraction of the muscles) at some point in their life.

It is important to realize that epilepsy is a neurological disorder—and not a disease. It is a condition produced by temporary changes in the brain, causing seizures that affect awareness, movement, or sensation. Medication controls the seizures in all but 30% or so of those affected. Alternatively, epileptics may require an implantable nerve stimulator or be forced to undergo surgical removal of brain tissue. Epilepsy kills 71,000 males and 55,000 females annually worldwide (World Health Organization 2005a).

Gamma Knife radiotherapy has been used throughout the world to treat epilepsy patients whose seizures are not controlled by medication. Treatment involves targeting the beam of radiation directly onto the temporal lobes—the region of the brain beneath the temples that is associated with memory, speech, and language. In France, a group reported achieving a significant improvement in overall quality of life noting that 65% of those irradiated with 24 Gy were seizure free after 2 years with only a few complaints of occasional depression, headache, and nausea (Regis et al. 2004).

Giant Cell Tumor

Giant cell tumors are benign tumors that account for as much as 10% of all primary bone tumors. They are more common in women than men and usually affect ages 25 to 40 years. The tumors are locally aggressive and removed by surgery. However, exposure to radiation can cause them to become malignant and metastasize to the lung. Also, there is a 50% probability of local tumor recurrence (Goh, Peh, and Shek 2002).

Radiotherapy after surgery has been used successfully at the New York University Medical Center to treat giant cell tumor of the spine in cases, where the tumor cannot be completely removed or where it results in severe functional morbidity (Khan et al. 1999). According to the University of Florida College of Medicine in Gainesville, Florida, lesions that are surgically inaccessible can be treated with up to 50 Gy EBRT to provide 65% to 80% local tumor control (Mendenhall et al. 2006).

Hyperthyroidism and Hypothyroidism

Exposing the thyroid gland to ionizing radiation is not without risk. Besides possibly causing thyroid cancer as discussed earlier, prior radiation exposure via radioiodine therapy or EBRT has also been linked to hypothyroidism and Graves' disease, the most common form of hyperthyroidism. The former is a condition in which there is a deficient production of thyroid hormones and the latter is an overproduction of thyroid hormones in which the patient's metabolism can increase 60% to 100% and can develop characteristically bulging eyeballs:

> Primary hypothyroidism, the most common radiation-induced thyroid dysfunction, affects 20-30% of patients administered following curative radiotherapy to the neck region, with approximately half of the events occurring within the first 5 years after therapy. (Jereczek-Fossa et al. 2004)

For obvious reasons, radiotherapy has no therapeutic value in treating hypothyroidism and so the treatment of choice is a thyroid hormone preparation. This procedure runs the risk of causing a heart attack or developing osteoporosis in post-menopausal women if over-prescribed (Clarke and Kabadi 2004).

Ironically, according to a group in Switzerland, the radioactive iodine treatment is most often prescribed for hyperthyroid patients, a procedure that is complicated because of the well-established "inverse correlation of pretherapeutic iodine uptake level and post-therapeutic outcome" in which 60% of the patients are cured, 20% remain in a hyperthyroid state, and 20% become hypothyroid (Walter et al. 2004).

But that is not the only concern. A Swedish study of 187 hyperthyroid patients treated with radioiodine concluded that on average, patients received more than twice the recommended dose with individual patients receiving up to eight times higher doses necessitating longer hospital stays and lengthier restrictions on patient exposure to family members (Jönsson and Mattson 2004).

Trigeminal Neuralgia

Trigeminal neuralgia is a non-fatal neurological disorder affecting the trigeminal nerve—the major sensory nerve of the face. More common in women than in men, trigeminal neuralgia is arguably the most painful affliction known to medical practitioners causing electric shock-like sensations that are triggered by talking and eating.

Although radiotherapy is not curative for this disorder, it offers palliative relief. For example, the University of Maryland Medical Center reported that initial (75 Gy) and repeat (70 Gy) SRS of refractory or recurrent trigeminal neuralgia patients

> resulted in a median 60% improvement in quality of life, and 56% of patients believed that the procedure was successful.... None of the 3 patients with pain refractory to initial [SRS] responded to repeat [treatment]. (Herman et al. 2004)

The Mayo Clinic prospectively compared the efficacy of SRS concluding that it is as cost-effective as conventional surgery but significantly less so than another popular treatment option—percutaneous glycerol rhizotomy (intentionally injuring the trigeminal nerve with an injection of glycerol—an alcohol found in wine). However, in terms of relieving pain for an extended time period, conventional surgery was noted as by far and away the preferred methodology (Pollock and Ecker 2005).

Vascular Malformations

The abnormal development of blood vessels in the CNS can lead to a web-like entanglement of arteries and veins called an arteriovenous malformation (AVM). AVMs are congenital disorders that are believed to affect 300,000 Americans although the symptoms of headaches, hemorrhaging (bleeding), and seizures (sudden involuntary muscle movement) are far less reaching. Usually not diagnosed in the first 20 years of life, AVMs can grow to more than 2 inches in diameter and are thought to account for some 2% of all hemorrhagic strokes, which of course can be fatal (National Institute of Neurological Disorders and Stroke 2006).

The Mayo Clinic in Rochester, Minnesota demonstrated some success in treating 56 AVM patients with radiosurgery between 1990 and 2000 obliterating the lesion in 39% and 48% of the patients after one or more procedures respectively and thus preventing any future risk of hemorrhage or death (Pollock, Gorman, and Brown 2004).

A more general collection of abnormal blood vessels that are not necessarily congenital and which are located anywhere in the body is called a cavernous malformation (CM). Accounting for some 15% of all venous malformations, most CMs are clinically insignificant. However, if this grouping of thin walled blood vessels is located in the brain it can cause seizures.

A recent Chinese study reported successfully treating 43 surgically high-risk CM patients with Gamma Knife radiosurgery achieving 28% seizure-freedom. In nine patients, however, rebleeding was confirmed and one died (Liu et al. 2005). In the United States, propitious outcomes with 16 cavernous malfunctions treated with surgery at the Louisiana State University Health Sciences Center were reviewed after a 5-year follow-up period (Berk et al. 2005).

Appendix

Institutions

Albert Einstein College of Medicine of Yeshiva University in New York City is one of six NCI-designated Cancer Centers in New York state.

Baylor College of Medicine, Houston, Texas, was founded in 1900 and is affiliated with seven hospitals.

Brigham and Women's Hospital in Boston, Massachusetts is the 27th best cancer hospital in the United States (U.S. News and World Report 2006).

City of Hope National Medical Center, Duarte, California is a NCI-designated Comprehensive Cancer Center and was ranked 43rd best cancer hospital in the United States (U.S. News and World Report 2005).

College of Physicians and Surgeons, Columbia University, New York, New York includes the NCI-designated Herbert Irving Comprehensive Cancer Center.

Dana-Farber Cancer Institute in Boston, Massachusetts is affiliated with Harvard Medical School. The state's only NCI-designated Comprehensive Cancer Center, it employs some 3000 people and treats upwards of 150,000 people per year. It is ranked 5th best cancer hospital in the United States (U.S. News and World Report 2006).

Duke Comprehensive Cancer Center in Durham, North Carolina is ranked 7th in the United States for cancer care and best in the Southeast (U.S. News and World Report 2006).

Duluth Community Clinical Oncology Program in Minnesota is one of a number of NCI sponsored endeavors providing clinical trial studies at a community based level.

Emory University Hospital, Atlanta, Georgia, is a 579-bed facility staffed exclusively by 800 Emory University School of Medicine faculty.

Fox Chase Cancer Center in Philadelphia is a NCI-designated Comprehensive Cancer Center and is ranked 16th best hospital in the United States (U.S. News and World Report 2006).

Fred Hutchinson Cancer Research Center is a non-profit organization located in Seattle, Washington that is known for its pioneering stem cell work. It is the only NCI-designated (Comprehensive) Cancer Center in the state.

Georgetown University Medical Center in Washington D.C. and its Lombardi Cancer Research Center is the only NCI-designated (Comprehensive) Cancer Center in the U.S. capital.

Harvard University, established in 1636 in Boston, Massachusetts now employes 9000 medical school faculty. The University has an endowment fund of $26 billion asnd has produced 43 Nobel Laureates.

Hoag Memorial Hospital Presbyterian in Newport Beach, California is a 511-bed, not-for-profit facility that is home to more than 1000 physicians.

Holy Name Hospital in Teaneck, New Jersey is a 361-bed facility and an academic affiliate of New York City's College of Physicians and Surgeons, Columbia University.

Hospital of the University of Pennsylvania, Philadelphia is ranked 27th best hospital in the United States by *U.S. News and World Report, 2005* and the affiliated Abramson Cancer Center is an NCI-designated Comprehensive Cancer Center.

Indiana University Cancer Center in Indianapolis is one of two NCI-designated cancer centers in Indiana. The center includes the Midwest Proton Radiotherapy Institute.

Johns Hopkins Hospital in Baltimore, Maryland is the only NCI-designated (Comprehensive) Cancer Center in the state and is ranked 3rd best hospital in the United States (U.S. News and World Report 2005, 2006).

Loma Linda University and Medical Center, in Loma Linda, California is a Seventh-day Adventist Institution that opened in 1967. It features a 900 bed children's hospital and the first proton treatment center in the United States.

Louisiana State University Health Sciences Center in Shreveport, Louisiana is a public institution founded in 1931.

Massachusetts General Hospital in Boston is ranked 15th best hospital in the United States (U.S. News and World Report 2006). The Francis H. Burr Proton Therapy Center is located on the main hospital campus.

Mayo Clinic in Rochester, Minnesota is one of two NCI-designated Comprehensive Cancer Centers in Minnesota and ranked 4th best hospital in the United States (U.S. News and World Report 2006).

Medical University of South Carolina in Charleston, South Carolina is a statewide consortium of teaching hospitals and rural health education centers.

Memorial Sloan-Kettering Cancer Center is located in New York. Founded in 1884, it is a NCI-designated Comprehensive Cancer Center and ranked as the best cancer hospital in the United States (U.S. News and World Report 2005, 2006).

H. Lee Moffitt Cancer Center and Research Institute in Tampa, Florida is the only NCI-designated (Comprehensive) Cancer Center in the state and is ranked 11th best hospital in the United States (U.S. News and World Report 2006).

Mount Sinai Medical Center was founded in 1852, today providing New York City with a 1171-bed teaching hospital and a medical staff of 1800.

New York University Medical Center in New York City is a NCI-designated Cancer Center and was ranked 33rd best cancer hospital in the United States (U.S. News and World Report 2005).

Ohio State University James Cancer Hospital in Columbus, Ohio is a NCI-designated Comprehensive Cancer Center and ranked 21st best hospital in the United States (U.S. News and World Report 2006).

Saint Jude Children's Research Hospital in Memphis, Tennessee is a NCI-designated Cancer Center. Founded in 1962 by Danny Thomas (1914-1991) it is dedicated to finding cures for catastrophic childhood diseases and known for treating children from all over the world.

Saint Vincent's Comprehensive Cancer Center in New York City specializes in treating multiple myeloma and other cancers.

Seattle Prostate Institute in the state of Washington, established in 1997 by an independent group of physicians, has treated more than 5000 patients with brachytherapy.

Stanford Hospital and Clinics, Stanford, California is ranked 14th best hospital in the United States (U.S. News and World Report 2006) and is part of the Stanford University Medical Center.

Thomas Jefferson University Hospital in Philadelphia, Pennsylvania includes the NCI-designated Kimmel Cancer Center, one of five Centers in the state. It is ranked the 48th best cancer hospital in the United States (U.S. News and World Report 2006).

University of Alabama Hospital at Birmingham is a NCI-designated Comprehensive Cancer Center, the only center in the state, and is ranked 23rd best hospital in the United States (U.S. News and World Report 2006).

University Medical Center in Tucson, Arizona is a NCI-designated Comprehensive Cancer Center, the only center in the state, and was ranked the 21st best hospital in the United States (U.S. News and World Report 2005).

University of California, Davis in Sacramento, California is a NCI-designated Cancer Center.

University of California, Irvine operates the Chao Family Comprehensive Cancer Center, one of six NCI-designated Comprehensive Cancer Centers in California. The University's Medical Center is ranked the 31st best cancer hospital in the United States (U.S. News and World Report 2006).

University of California, Los Angeles (UCLA) Medical Center in Los Angeles, California is a NCI-designated Comprehensive Cancer Center and is ranked 9th best hospital in the United States (U.S. News and World Report 2006).

University of California, San Diego in La Jolla, California is a NCI-designated Comprehensive Cancer Center. The University's Medical Center is ranked the 33rd best cancer hospital in the United States (U.S. News and World Report 2006).

University of California, San Francisco Medical Center is a NCI-designated Comprehensive Cancer Center and is ranked 10th best cancer hospital in the United States (U.S. News and World Report 2006).

University of Chicago Hospitals is a NCI-designated Comprehensive Cancer Center and was ranked 8th best hospital in the United States (U.S. News and World Report 2006).

University of Colorado Cancer Center in Aurora, Colorado is the only NCI-designated (Comprehensive) Cancer Center in the state. The University's hospital in Denver is ranked 32nd best cancer hospital in the United States (U.S. News and World Report 2006).

University of Florida College of Medicine in Gainesville, Florida has produced more than 3700 physicians since graduating its first medical students in 1960.

University of Florida's Shands Medical Center in Jacksonville, Florida includes nine hospitals and features a proton beam cancer treatment facility.

University Hospitals of Cleveland is ranked 13th best cancer hospital in the United States (U.S. News and World Report 2006) and is affiliated with the Case Western Reserve University cancer center in Cleveland, one of two NCI-designated Comprehensive Cancer Centers in Ohio.

University of Maryland Medical Center in Baltimore is a teaching hospital serving more than 250,000 patients annually.

University of Miami Miller School of Medicine in Florida opened in 1952 and now treats more than one million patients annually and from as far away as South America.

University of Michigan Medical Center in Ann Arbor, Michigan is a NCI-designated Comprehensive Cancer Center and ranked 18th best cancer hospital in the United States (U.S. News and World Report 2006).

University of North Carolina at Chapel Hill is one of three NCI-designated Comprehensive Cancer Centers in the state of North Carolina. The university's hospital is ranked the 40th best cancer hospital in the United States (U.S. News and World Report 2006).

University of Pittsburgh Medical Center is a NCI-designated Comprehensive Cancer Center and is ranked 12th best hospital in the United States (U.S. News and World Report 2006).

University of Southern California is one of the two NCI-designated Comprehensive Cancer Centers in Los Angeles, California.

University of Texas, M. D. Anderson Cancer Center in Houston, Texas was established in 1941. It is a NCI-designated Comprehensive Cancer Center, one of two centers in the state, and is ranked 2nd best cancer hospital in the United States (U.S. News and World Report 2005, 2006). The **M. D. Anderson Cancer Center Orlando**, an affiliate, opened in Orlando, Florida in 1991.

University of Utah Hospitals and Clinics in Salt Lake City, Utah is ranked 34th best hospital in the United States (U.S. News and World Report 2006). The university's Huntsman Cancer Institute is the state's only NCI-designated Cancer Center.

University of Virginia Medical Center, Charlottesville is one of two NCI-designated Cancer Centers in Virginia and is ranked

30th best hospital in the United States (U.S. News and World Report 2006).

University of Washington Medical Center, in Seattle is ranked 6th best hospital in the United States (U.S. News and World Report 2006).

University of Wisconsin Hospital and Clinics, Madison, Wisconsin is ranked 28th best hospital in the United States (U.S. News and World Report 2005, 2006) and serves as a NCI-designated Comprehensive Cancer Center.

Washington Hospital Center was founded in 1958 and is today the largest cancer care provider in Washington D.C. having diagnosed more than 2600 new cases in 2005.

Washington University School of Medicine in Saint Louis, Missouri includes the Alvin J. Siteman Cancer Center, the Mallinckrodt Institute of Radiology, and the Barnes-Jewish Hospital, ranked 17th best cancer hospital in the United States (U.S. News and World Report 2006).

Wayne State University in Detroit, Michigan is one of the state's two NCI-designated Comprehensive Cancer Centers.

Yale-New Haven Medical Center in New Haven, Connecticut is a NCI-designated Comprehensive Cancer Center, the only center in the state, and is ranked 26th best hospital in the United States (U.S. News and World Report 2006).

Organizations

American Cancer Society (ACS), founded in 1913, is a charitable organization in the United States that funds cancer research, second only to the federal government in money spent dedicated to eliminating cancer.

American College of Physicians (ACP), founded in 1915, is with nearly 120,000 members, the largest medical-specialty organization in the United States.

American College of Radiology is a 30,000-member professional organization that offers various classes of membership to people working in the medicine-radiation field.

California Cancer Registry is a U.S. statewide population-based cancer surveillance system that today has collected detailed information on over 1.3 million cases of cancer.

Canadian Task Force on Preventive Health Care, formerly known as the Canadian Task Force on the Periodic Health Examination, was established in 1976 and is funded by the government to make health recommendations.

Centers for Disease Control and Prevention (CDC), founded in 1946, is an agency of the U.S. Department of Health and Human Services. CDC's 9000 employees are chartered with preventing disease, injury, and disability of all people in all communities.

Fermi National Accelerator Laboratory (Fermilab) in Batavia, Illinois is a national laboratory of the U.S. government founded in 1967 and in 1974 named after Enrico Fermi (1901-1954), the very special Nobel winning radiation physicist, who died of stomach cancer.

Food and Drug Administration (FDA) is an agency of the U.S. Department of Health and Human Services chartered with regulating food and drug consumption and medical device products.

Health Physics Society is a 6,000-member organization of professionals founded in 1956 that is devoted to radiation safety awareness.

Leukaemia Research is a charitable organization established in 1960 devoted to serving lymphatic cancer patients in the U.K.

The Leukemia & Lymphoma Society was founded in 1949 and is today the world's largest voluntary organization dedicated to curing blood cancers.

National Academy of Sciences is a corporation that since 1863 has made recommendations on science, engineering, and medicine to the U.S. government. Boasting 170 plus Nobel Laureates, election to the Academy is one of the highest honors given a scientist.

National Association for Proton Therapy is a non-profit organization in the United States founded in 1990 and chartered with promoting the advantages of proton therapy for cancer treatment.

National Cancer Institute (NCI), established in 1937, is one of the 27 Institutes and Centers under the U.S. Department of Health and Human Services. NCI sponsors 39 Comprehensive Cancer Centers that integrate laboratory, clinical and population-based research, and 22 Cancer Centers that focus on basic, population sciences, or clinical research, or any two of the three, as of April 2006.

National Cancer Institute of Canada (NCIC) was formed in 1947 to reduce in Canada, incidence, morbidity, and mortality from cancer.

National Familial Pancreas Cancer Registry (NFPCR) was established at Johns Hopkins University, Maryland, in 1994 to assist in the diagnosis and treatment of pancreatic cancer.

National Institute of Diabetes and Digestive and Kidney Diseases (NIDDK), established in 1948, is one of the 27 Institutes and Centers under the U.S. Department of Health and Human Services. NIIDDK researches a broad spectrum of metabolic diseases affecting public health.

National Institute of Environmental Health Sciences (NIEHS), established in 1969, is one of the 27 Institutes and Centers under the U.S. Department of Health and Human Services. NIEHS supports the National Toxicology Program, established in 1978, to fund university research and evaluate the testing of harmful chemicals and other substances.

National Institute of Neurological Disorders and Stroke (NINDS), created in 1950, is one of the 27 Institutes and Centers under the U.S. Department of Health and Human Services. NINDS conducts research on Parkinson's disease, stroke, and epilepsy.

National Institute for Occupational Safety and Health (NIOSH), created in 1970, is an agency of the U.S. Department of Health and Human Services. NIOSH provides research and recommends work-related illness, injury and disability measures.

National Research Council of Canada (NRC) founded in 1916 is the Canadian government's largest R&D organization. It is composed of over 20 institutes and national programs employing 4000 people.

National Society for Epilepsy (NSE) is the largest epileptic charity in the U.K. providing medical assistance since 1892.

National Surgical Adjuvant Breast and Bowel Project, headquartered in Pittsburgh, Pennsylvania, is a NCI sponsored clinical trials group representing the United States, Canada, Puerto Rico, and Australia.

National Toxicology Program (NTP) has the same director as the National Institute of Environmental Health and Sciences, but reports on NTP matters to the U.S. Department of Health and Human Services.

Oak Ridge National Laboratory (ONRL) in Tennessee is a giant 58 square mile facility operated by the U.S. Department of

Energy that provides the medical community with a number of radioisotopes including californium-252.

Radiation Effects Research Foundation in Japan is a joint Japanese-American organization that studies the effects of radiation on survivors of the 1945 Hiroshima and Nagasaki atomic bombings.

U.S. Department of Health and Human Services (HHS) is a department of the United States established in 1953 and given a 2006 budget of $573.5 billion (mandatory) and $67.2 billion (discretionary) intended to protect the health of all Americans.

U.S. Environmental Protection Agency (EPA) is a government agency, established in 1970, chartered with protecting human health and safeguarding the environment.

U.S. Preventive Services Task Force is an independent panel of medical experts that since 1984 has made recommendations for primary care.

World Health Organization (WHO) is the United Nations health agency, established in 1948, and headquartered in Geneva, Switzerland, chartered with combating disease worldwide.

Glossary

ablation (*ah-BLAY-shun*): removal of a surface with intense energy.

adenocarcinoma (*A-de-no-kar-si-NO-ma*): a cancer that originates in cells that line certain internal organs.

adjunctive (*ad-JUNK-tive*): see **adjuvant**.

adjuvant (*Aj-e-vent*): additional treatment used to increase the effectiveness of the primary therapy.

anaplasia (*an-ah-PLAY-zha*): the appearance of non-normal cells that have no structure are named **anaplastic** (*an-ah-PLAS-tik*) cells.

angiography (*AN-jee-OG-ra_fee*): a diagnostic tool that uses specialized dyes to highlight X-ray or other images.

benign (*bee-NINE*): not cancerous.

brachytherapy (*BRACK-ee-ther-a-pee*): internal radiation therapy.

carcinoid (*KAR-sin-oyd*): a slow-growing tumor usually associated with the gastrointestinal tract.

carcinogenic (*kar-sin-oh-JEN-ic*): cancer causing.

carcinoma (*kar-si-NO-ma*): the most common type of cancer and which arise from the epithelial cells.

cisplatin (SIS-pla-tun): an anticancer drug that enhances radiotherapy; also called Platinol®.

congenital (*kon-JENi-tal*): a condition existing from birth.

cystoscopy (sist-OSS-ko-pee): visual examination and treatment of urinary tract problems with an external probe.

deoxyribonucleic acid (dee-ok-see-ri-bo-new-CLAY-ic): organic material in every cell and certain viruses that carries the genetic code; abbreviated DNA.

duodenum (*doo-ah-DEE-num*): the first part of the small intestine nearest to the stomach.

enzyme (*EN-zime*): proteins that speed up chemical reactions in the body.

epithelial (*ep-i-THEE-lee-ul*): cells that line a surface and define its boundary.

glioma (*glee-O-ma*): a non-metastatic tumor of the brain and spinal cord that does not originate from nerve cells.

hematopoiesis (*hee-ma-to-poi-asis*): formation of blood cells.

hyperplasia (*hye-per-PLAY-zha*): an abnormal increase in the number of cells in an organ or tissue that is not cancerous.

immunosuppression (*im-mune-no-suh-PREH-shun*): the less than normal ability of the body to fight disease that may exist from birth or develop later.

indolent (*IN-doe-lint*): a slow growing cancer.

Interferon (in-tur-feeR-on): a protein produced by white blood cells to fight viral infections.

lesion (*lee-zhun*): an abnormal structure in the body also an injury or wound.

linac (*LYNN-ack*): a machine that uses electricity to create high-energy radiation.

lymph (limf): nodes or glands or tissue that make up the immune system and fight infection; produce the white blood cells that fight disease.

lymphadenopathy (lim-fa-de-no-pathy): affecting lymph node(s).

malignant (*ma-o-aj-e-vent*): cancerous.

metastasis (*meh-TAS-ta-sis*): the spread of cancer to another part of the body; **metastases** (*meh-TAS-ta-ses*) is plural.

nasopharyngeal (NA-zoh-fuh-RIN-jee-ul): the upper part of the throat directly behind the nose.

neoadjuvant (*ne-o-aj-e-vent*): therapy administered prior to another therapy.

neoplasia (*NEE-oh-PLAY-zha*): abnormal and uncontrolled cell growth resulting in a tumor.

neuroma (*nur-oh-ma*): a non-cancerous tumor that originates in nerve cells.

oncogenic (*on-ko-JEN-ik*): a cancer causing physiological process or virus.

oncologist (*on-KAHL-o-jist*): a medical doctor who specializes in **oncology** (*on-KAHL-o-gee*), the study and treatment of cancer.

palliative (*pa-LEE-a-tive*): therapy intended to provide pain relief and deemed unlikely to extend life.

papillomavirus (*pap-ih-LO-ma-VYE-rus*): a virus that causes warts and now listed as a carcinogen.

pathogen (PATH-oh-jen): collectively refers to any bacteria, virus, protozoa, fungi or parasite that causes disease

photon (*Fo-ton*): smallest unit of X-ray and gamma ray radiation; also of ultraviolet, visible and infrared light.

platelets (*plAt-lits*): small, disc shaped cells in the blood that promote clotting.

pleural (*PLOOR-al*): relating to the pleura, the thin lubricating tissue covering the lungs.

precancerous (*pre-KAN-ser-us*): a condition likely to become malignant.

prognosis (*prog-NO-sis*): the expected way a disease will turn out.

radiation (*ray-dee-AY-shun*): the transmission or spread of energy.

refractory (*ree-frak-taree*): a cancer that does not respond to treatment.

remission (*ree-mi-shun*): partial or complete decrease in cancer symptoms with the cancer still present.

sarcoma (*Sar-kow-mu*): a cancer originating from connective tissue, such as muscle, fat, cartilage, and bone.

squamous (SKWA-muhs): cells of the skin.

syndrome (*sin-drohm*): a group or pattern of symptoms.

systemic (*sis-TEM-ik*): affecting all cells of the body.

tamoxifen (ta-MOK-si-FEN): an antibreast cancer drug.

vascular (VAS-ku-lar): anything having to do with blood vessels.

Bibliography

Abbott, B.L. Chronic lymphocytic leukemia: recent advances in diagnosis and treatment. The Oncologist 11 (2006): 21-30.

Ahamad, A. et al. Promising early local control of malignant pleural mesothelioma following postoperative intensity modulated radiotherapy (IMRT) to the chest. Cancer J. 9 (2003): 476-484.

Al-Hilli, F. and Ansari, N.A. Metastatic malignancies of unknown primary site and malignancies of unknown origin whether primary or metastatic. Saudi Med. J. 26 (2005): 1840-1843.

Ali, M. The clinical value of the PSA test for assessing prostate health and managing cancer, posted 28 February 2005. <http://www.majidali.com/psa_clinical_value_prostate_cancer.htm> (7 April 2006).

Allolio, B. and Fassnacht, M. Adrenocorticol carcinoma: clinical update. J. Clin. Endocrinol. Metab. 91 (2006): 2027-2037.

American Cancer Society. ACS 2005 fact sheet, revised January 2005a. <http://www.cancer.org/docroot/AA/content/AA_1_2_ACS_Fact_Sheet.asp> (20 April 2006).

American Cancer Society, interview by TheBostonChannel.com. Researchers suggest cutting back on steak, chops. TheBostonChannel.com. 11 January 2005b. <http://www.thebostonchannel.com/health/4072657/detail.html> (12 January 2006).

American Cancer Society. What are the key statistics about laryngeal and hypopharyngeal cancers? revised 16 December 2005c. <http://www.cancer.org/docroot/cri/content/cri_2_4_1x_what_are_the_key_statistics_for_laryngeal_and_hypopharyngeal_cancer_23.asp?sitearea=&level=> (6 June 2006).

American Cancer Society. American Cancer Society report finds drop in total cancer deaths, posted 9 February 2006a. <http://www.cancer.org/docroot/MED/content/MED_2_1x_American_Cancer_Society_Report_Finds_Drop_in_Total_Cancer_Deaths.asp> (1 June 2006).

American Cancer Society. Radiation exposure and cancer, revised 6 February 2006b. <http://www.cancer.org/docroot/PED/content/PED_1_3X_Radiation_Exposure_and_Cancer.asp?> (27 May 2006).

American Cancer Society. Statistics for 2006, posted 2006c. <http://www.cancer.org/docroot/STT/stt_0.asp> (31 May 2006).

American Cancer Society. What are the key statistics about thymus cancers? revised 23 January 2006d. <http://www.cancer.org/docroot/CRI/content/CRI_2_4_1X_What_ar e_the_key_statistics_for_thymus_cancer_42.asp?sitearea=> (12 June 2006).

American Cancer Society. What are the key statistics for Wilms tumor? revised 12 February 2006e. <http://www.cancer.org/docroot/CRI/content/CRI_2_4_1X_What_ar e_the_key_statistics_for_Wilms_tumor_46.asp?sitearea=> (6 June 2006).

American Cancer Society. What are the risk factors for brain and spinal cord tumors in adults? revised 10 March 2006f. <http://www.cancer.org/docroot/CRI/content/CRI_2_4_2X_What_ar e_the_risk_factors_for_brain_and_spinal_cord_tumors_3.asp?sitear ea=> (11 April 2006).

American College of Physicians. Arguments against aggressive treatment, posted 15 March 1997. <http://www.prostatepointers.org/ww/notreat.htm> (2 June 2006).

American Shared Hospital Services. Gamma Knife, updated 1 June 2006. <http://www.ashs.com/gammaknife.htm> (19 June 2006).

American Society of Plastic Surgeons. 2000/2004/2005 National plastic surgery statistics, posted 2006. <http://www.plasticsurgery.org/public_education/loader.cfm?url=/co mmonspot/security/getfile.cfm&PageID=17870> (15 June 2006).

Amundadottir, L.T. et al. Cancer as a complex phenotype: pattern of cancer distribution within and beyond the nuclear family. PLoS Med. 1 (2004): 229-236.

Albertsson, M. Chemoradiotherapy of esophageal cancer. Acta Oncologica 41 (2002): 118-123.

Almahroos, M. and Kurban A.K. Ultraviolet carcinogenesis in nonmelanoma skin cancer. Part I: incidence rate in relation to geographic location and in migrant populations. Skinmed. 3 (2004): 29-35.

Ando, T. et al. Causal role of Helicobacter pylori infection in gastric cancer. World J. Gastroenterol. 12 (2006): 181-186.

Andres, A. Cancer incidence after immunosuppressive treatment following kidney transplantation. Crit. Rev. Oncol. Hematol. 56 (2005): 71-85.

Ansell, S.M. and Armitage, J.O. Management of Hodgkin lymphoma. Mayo Clin. Proc. 3 (2006): 419-426.

Arafah, B.M. and Nasrallah, M.P. Pituitary tumors: pathophysiology, clinical manifestations and management. Endocrine-Related Cancer 8 (2001): 287-305.

Ardeshna, K.M. et al. Long-term effect of a watch and wait policy versus immediate systemic treatment for asymptomatic advanced-stage non-Hodgkin lymphoma: a randomised controlled trial. Lancet 362 (2003): 516-522.

Arnold, R. et al. Unrelated bone marrow transplantation in patients with myelodysplastic syndromes and secondary acute myeloid leukemia: an EBMT survey. European Blood and Marrow Transplantation Group. Bone Marrow Transplant 21 (1998): 1213-1216.

Aul, C., Bowen, D.T. and Yoshida, Y. Pathogenesis, etiology and epidemiology of myeloplastic syndromes. Haematologica 83 (1998): 71-86.

Ault, K.A. Vaccines for the prevention of human papillomavirus and associated gynecologic diseases: a review. Obstet. Gynecol. Surv. 61 (2006): S26-31.

Aupérin, A. et al. Prophylactic cranial irradiation for patients with small-cell lung cancer in complete remission. N. Engl. J. Med. 341 (1999): 476-484.

Avril, M.F. et al. Fotemustine compared with decarbazine in patients with disseminated malignant melanoma: a phase III study. J. Clin. Oncol. 22 (2004): 1118-1125.

Ayhan, A. et al. The long-term survival of women with surgical stage II endometroid type endometrial cancer. Gynecol. Oncol. 93 (2004): 9-13.

Aziz, T., Jilaihawi, A. and Prakash, D. 2002. The management of malignant pleural mesothelioma; single centre experience in 10 years. Eur. J. Cardiothorac. Surg. 22 (2002): 298-305.

Bacin, F. et al. Long-term results of cobalt 60 Curietherapy for uveal melanoma. J. Fr. Ophthalmol. 21 (1998): 333-344.

Baines, C.J. and Miller, A.B. Mammography versus clinical examination of the breasts. J. Natl. Cancer Inst. Monogr. 22 (1997): 125-129.

Bakai, A., Alber, M. and Nusslin, F. Estimation of a radiation time prolongation factor for intensity-modulated radiotherapy. Phys. Med. Biology 48 (2003): N25-29.

Bamias, A. et al. Adjuvant chemotherapy with paclitaxel and carboplatin in patients with advanced carcinoma of the upper urinary tract: a study by the Hellenic Cooperative Oncology Group. J. Clin. Oncol. 22 (2004): 2150-2154.

Baraua, K.K. et al. Treatment of recurrent craniopharyngiomas, Kobe J. Med. Sci., 49 (2003): 123-132.

Bardawil, T. and Manetta, A. Surgical treatment of vaginal cancer, updated 20 July 2005. <http://www.emedicine.com/med/topic3330.htm> (2 June 2006).

Baum, M., interview by Laura Barclay. Controversy rages over breast cancer screening: a newsmaker interview with Michael Baum, MD. Medscape Medical News, 3 September 2002.

Behari, A. et al. Longterm survival after extended resections in patients with gallbladder cancer. J. Am. Coll. Surg. 196 (2003): 82-88.

Benedetti-Panici, P. et al. Neoadjuvant chemotherapy and radical surgery versus exclusive radiotherapy in locally advanced squamous cell cervical cancer: results from the Italian Multicenter Randomized Study. J. Clin. Oncol. 20 (2002): 179-188.

Benke, K.K. Biological effects of low-level radiation and diagnostic medical X-rays. J. Australas. College Nutr. Environ. Med. 14 (1995): 17-20.

Berk, C. et al. Surgical management of intracranial cavernous malformations: the Louisiana State University Health Sciences Center, Shreveport experience. South Med. J. 98 (2005): 611-615.

Berrington de Gonzalez, A. and Darby, S. Risk of cancer from diagnostic X-rays: estimates for the UK and 14 other countries. Lanclet 363 (2004): 345-351.

Biasco, G. et al. Treatment of hepatic metastases from colorectal cancer: many doubts, some certainties. Cancer Treat Rev. 32 (2006): 214-228.

Bielack, S.S. et al. Prognostic factors in high-grade osteosarcoma of the extremeties or trunk: an analysis of 1,702 patients treated on neoadjuvant cooperative osteosarcoma study group protocols. J. Clin. Oncol. 20 (2002): 776-790.

Bilsky, M.H. et al. Intensity-modulated stereotactic radiotherapy of paraspinal tumors: a preliminary report. Neurosurg. 54 (2004): 823-830.

Bjork-Eriksson, T. and Glimelius, B. The potential of proton beam radiation therapy in breast cancer. Acta Oncol. 44 (2005): 844-849.

Blair, A. et al. Immunotherapeutic strategies in acute lymphoblastic leukaemia relapsing after stem cell transplantation. Blood Rev. 19 (2005): 289-300.

Blasko, J.C. et al. The role of external beam radiotherapy with I-125/Pd-103 brachytherapy for prostate carcinoma. Radiother. Oncol. 57 (2000): 273-278.

Blom, D. and Schwartz, S.I. Surgical treatment and outcomes in carcinoma of the extrahepatic bile ducts: the University of Rochester experience. Arch. Surg. 136 (2001): 209-215.

Boffetta, P. et al. Meta-analysis of studies of occupational exposure to vinyl chloride in relation to cancer mortality. Scand. J. Work Environ. Health. 3 (2003): 220-229.

Bogardus, C.R., Jr. Is IMRT cost effective for your center. Oncology Issues 15 (2000): 11-14.

Bogardus, C.R., Jr. Economic issues related to IMRT. Oncology Issues 18 (2003a): 4-6.

Bogardus, C.R., Jr. IMRT: an overview. Oncology Issues 18 Suppl. 2 (2003b): 5-7.

Boice, J.D., Jr. Cancer following medical irradiation. Cancer 47 (1981): 1081-1090.

Boice, J.D., Jr. and Miller, R.W. Childhood and adult cancer after intrauterine exposure to ionizing radiation. Teratology 59 (1999): 227-233.

Bokemeyer, C. et al. Extragonadal germ cell tumors: relation to testicular neoplasia and management options. Acta Pathol. Microbiol. Immunol. Scand. 111 (2003): 49-59.

Borchardt, P.E. et al. Targeted actinium-225 in vivo generators for therapy of ovarian cancer. Cancer Res. 63 (2003): 5084-5090.

Bosetti, C. et al. Occupational exposure to vinyl chloride and cancer risk: a review of the epidemiologic literature. Eur. J. Cancer Prev. 12 (2003): 427-430.

Boucher, E. et al. Adjuvant intra-arterial injection of iodine-131-labeled lipiodol after resection of hepatocellular carcinoma. Hepatology 38 (2003): 1237-1241.

Breitfeld, P.P. and Meyer, W.H. Rhabdomosarcoma: new windows of opportunity. Oncologist 10 (2005): 518-527.

Breitz, H. et al. Dosimetry of high dose skeletal targeted radiotherapy (STR) with 166Ho-DOTMP. Cancer Biother. Radiopharm. 18 (2003): 225-230.

Brenn, T. and Fletcher, C.D. Postradiation vascular proliferations: an increasing problem. Histopathology 48 (2006): 106-114.

Brenner, D.J. et al. Second malignancies in prostate carcinoma patients after radiotherapy compared with surgery. 88 (2000): 398-406.

Brenner, D.J. et al. Estimated risks of radiation-induced fetal cancer from pediatric CT. Am. J. Roentgenology 176 (2001): 289-296.

Brenner, D.J. Estimating cancer risks from pediatric CT: going from the qualitative to the quantitative. Pediatric Radiol. 32 (2002): 228-231.

Brenner, D.J. et al. Routine screening mammography: how important is the radiation-risk side of the benefit-risk equation? Int. J. Radiat. Bio. 78 (2002): 1065-1067.

Brenner, D.J. Radiation risks potentially associated with low-dose CT screening of adult smokers for lung cancer. Radiology 231 (2004): 440-445.

Breslow, N. et al. Epidemiology of Wilms tumor. Med. Pediatr. Oncol. 21 (1993): 172-181.

Brewster, W.R. et al. Intent-to-treat analysis of stage Ib and IIa cervical cancer in the United States: radiotherapy or surgery 1988-1995. Obstet. Gynecol. 97 (2001): 248-254.

Brierley, J.D. and Tsang, R.W. External-beam radiation therapy in the treatment of differentiated thyroid cancer. Semin. Surg. Oncol. 16 (1999): 42-49.

British Council. Health insight May 2001: new British research. <http://www.britishcouncil.org/health/themes/insight/may01/research.htm> (29 March 2004).

Brookhaven National Laboratory. The technetium-99m generator, no date. <http://www.bnl.gov/bnlweb/history/Tc-99m.asp> (10 June 2004).

Brown, M.L. et al. Estimating health care costs related to cancer treatment from SEER-Medicare data. Medical Care 40 Suppl. 8 (2002): IV-104-107.

Buadi, F.K. et al. Autolgous hematopoietic stem-cell transplantation for older patients with relapsed non-Hodgkin's lymphoma. Bone Marrow Transplant. 37 (2006): 1017-1022.

Buchholz, T.A. et al. The role of fast neutron radiation therapy in the management of advanced salivary gland malignant neoplasms. Cancer 69 (1992): 2779-2788.

Burke, J.M., Jurcic, J.G. and Scheinberg, D.A. Radioimmunotherapy for acute leukemia. Cancer Control 9 (2002): 106-113.

Campbell, S.C., Flanigan, R.C. and Clark, J.I. Nephrectomy in metastatic renal cell carcinoma. Curr. Treat. Options Oncol. 4 (2003): 363-372.

Cameron, J.H. Are X-rays safe? updated 22 May 1998. <http://www.angelfire.com/mo/radioadaptive/jcameron1.html> (31 March 2004).

Cameron, J.L. et al. Management of proximal cholangiocarcinomas by surgical resection and radiotherapy. Am. J. Surg. 59 (1990): 91-97.

Canadian Cancer Society. Canadian cancer statistics 2006, posted 2006. <http://129.33.170.32/vgn/images/portal/cit_86751114/31/21/93550 5792cw_2006stats_en.pdf.pdf> (8 June 2006).

Cancer Research UK. CancerStats, updated May 2006. <http://info.cancerresearchuk.org/cancerstats/> (6 June 2006).

Carbone, M. and Rdzanek, M.A. Pathogenesis of malignant mesothelioma. Clin. Lung Cancer 5 (2004): S46-S50.

Carter, J. and Pather, S. An overview of uterine cancer and its management. Expert Rev. Anticancer Ther. 6 (2006): 33-42.

Castellsague, X. et al. The role of type of tobacco and type of alcoholic beverage in oral carcinogenesis. Int. J. Cancer 108 (2004): 741-749.

Cattelan, A.M., Trevenzoli, M. and Aversa, S.M. Recent advances in the treatment of AIDS-related Kaposi's sarcoma. Am. J. Clin. Dermatol. 3 (2002): 451-462.

Centers for Disease Control and Prevention. Cancer survivorship, posted 25 June 2004a. <http://www.cdc.gov/mmwr/preview/mmwrhtml/mm5324a3.htm> (2 June 2006).

Centers for Disease Control and Prevention. NIOSH carcinogen list, reviewed 29 September 2004b. <http://www.cdc.gov/niosh/npotocca.html> (10 April 10 2006).

Centers for Disease Control and Prevention. Facts about benzene, reviewed 22 February 2006a. http://www.bt.cdc.gov/agent/benzene/basics/facts.asp> (16 June 2006).

Centers for Disease Control and Prevention. Mammography, reviewed 8 May 2006b. <http://www.cdc.gov/nchs/fastats/mamogram.htm> (13 June 2006).

Centers for Disease Control and Prevention, CDC's advisory committee recommends human papillomavirus vaccination. 29 June 2006c. <http://www.cdc.gov/od/oc/media/pressrel/r060629.htm> (30 June 2006).

Chahal, R. et al. A study of the morbidity, mortality and long-term survival following radical cystectomy and radical radiotherapy in the treatment of invasive bladder cancer in Yorkshire. Eur. Urol. 43 (2003): 246-257.

Chang, C.H. et al. Comparison of postoperative radiotherapy and combined postoperative radiotherapy and chemotherapy in the multidisciplinary management of malignant gliomas. A joint Radiation Therapy Oncology Group and Eastern Cooperative Oncology Group study. Cancer 52 (1993): 997-1007.

Chang, C.H. et al. Long-term results of hepatic resection for hepatocellular carcinoma originating from the noncirrhotic liver. Arch. Surg. 139 (2004): 320-325.

Chang, T-C. et al. Randomized trial of neoadjuvant cisplatin, vincristine, bleomycin, and radical hysterectomy versus radiation therapy for bulky stage IB and IIA cervical cancer. J. Clin. Oncol. 18 (2000): 1740-1747.

Chao, A. et al. Meat consumption and risk of colorectal cancer. J. Am. Med. Assoc. 293 (2005): 172-182.

Chen, M.F. et al. Contemporary management of penile cancer including surgery and adjuvant radiotherapy: an experience in Taiwan. World J. Urol. 22 (2004): 60-66.

Cheng, J.C. et al. Radiation-induced liver disease after three-dimensional conformal radiotherapy for patients with hepatocellular carcinoma; dosimetric analysis and implication. Int. J. Radiat. Oncol. Biol. Phys. 54 (2002): 156-162.

Cheok, M.H., Lugthart, S. and Evans, W.E. Pharmacogenomics of acute leukemia. Annu. Rev. Pharmacol. Toxicol. 46 (2006): 317-353.

Cheung, M.C., Pantanowitz and L. Dezube, B.J. AIDS-related malignancies: emerging challenges in the era of highly active antiretroviral therapy. The Oncologist. 10 (2005): 412-426.

Child, J.A. et al. High-dose chemotherapy with hematopoietic stem-cell rescue for multiple myeloma. N. Engl. J. Med. 348 (2003): 1875-1883.

Chronowski, G.M. et al. Analysis of in-field control and late toxicity for adults with early-stage Hodgkin's disease treated with chemotherapy followed by radiotherapy. Int. J. Radiat. Oncol. Biol. Phys. 55 (2003): 36-43.

Cirillo, R.L., Jr. Adrenal carcinoma, updated 1 March 2005. <http://www.emedicine.com/radio/topic14.htm> (2 June 2006).

Clamon, G.H. Management of primary mediastinal seminoma. Chest 83 (1983): 263-267.

Clark, C.H. et al. Intensity-modulated radiotherapy improves target coverage, spinal cord sparing and allows dose escalation in patients with locally advanced cancer of the larynx. Radiother. Oncol. 70 (2004): 189-198.

Clarke, N. and Kabadi, U.M. Optimizing treatment of hypothyroidism. Treat. Endocrinol. 3 (2004): 217-221.

Clayman, G.L. et al. Parathyroid carcinoma: evaluation and interdisciplinary management. Cancer 100 (2004): 900-905.

Coleman, R.E. Bisphosphonates: clinical experience. Oncologist Suppl. 4 (2004): 14-27.

Colls, B.M. et al. Bilateral germ cell testicular tumors in New Zealand: experience in Auckland and Christchurch 1978-1994. J. Clin. Oncol. 14 (1996): 2061-2065.

Colombo, N. et al. International Collaborative Ovarian Neoplasm Trial 1: a randomized trial of adjuvant chemotherapy in women with early-stage ovarian cancer. J. Natl. Cancer Inst. 95 (2003): 125-132.

Conlon, K.C., Klimstra, D.S. and Brennan, M.F. Long-term survival after curative resection for pancreatic ductal adenocarcinoma.

Clinicopathologic analysis of 5-year survivors. Ann. Surg. 223 (1996): 273-279.

Connors, J.M. State-of-the-art therapeutics: Hodgkin's lymphoma. 23 (2005): 6400-6408.

Cook, A.D., Single, R., and McCahill, L.E. Surgical resection of primary tumors in patients who present with stage IV colorectal cancer: an analysis of surveillance, epidemiology, and end results data, 1988 to 2000. Ann Surg Oncol. 12 (2005): 637-645.

Coppin, J. et al. Improved local control of invasive bladder cancer by concurrent cisplatin and preoperative or definitive radiation. The National Cancer Institute of Canada Clinical Trials Group. Clin. Oncol. 14 (1996): 2901-2907.

Cortes, J. and Kantarjian, H. New targeted approaches in chronic myeloid leukemia. J. Clin. Oncol. 23 (2005): 6316-6324.

Cotterill, S.J. et al. Clinical prognostic factors in 1277 patients with neuroblastoma: results of The European Neuroblastoma Study Group 'Survey' 1982-1992. Eur. J. Cancer 36 (2000): 901-908.

Cotton, P.B. et al. Computed tomographic colonography (virtual colonoscopy): a multicenter comparison with standard colonoscopy for detection of colorectal neoplasia. J. Am. Med. Assoc. 291 (2004): 1713-1719.

Crane, C.H. et al. Limitations of conventional doses of chemoradiation for unresectable biliary cancer. Int. J. Radiat. Oncol. Biol. Phys. 53 (2002): 969-974.

Creasman, W.T. Vaginal cancers. Curr. Opin. Obstet. Gynecol. 17 (2005): 71-76.

Cress, R.D. et al. Survival among patients with adenocarcinoma of the pancreas: a population-based study (United States). Cancer Causes Control 17 (2006): 403-409.

Crew, K.D. and Neugut, A.I. Epidemiology of gastric cancer. World J. Gastroenterol. 12 (2006): 354-362.

Creutzberg, C.L. et al. The morbidity of treatment for patients with stage I endometrial cancer: results from a randomized trial. Int. J. Radiat. Oncol. Biol. Phys. 51 (2001): 1246-1255.

Creutzberg, C.L. et al. Outcome of high-risk stage IC, grade 3, compared with stage I endometrial carcinoma patients: the postoperative radiation therapy in endometrial carcinoma trial. J. Clin. Oncol. 22 (2004): 1234-1241.

Cripe, T.P. Rhabdomyosarcoma, updated 7 October 2006. <http://www.emedicine.com/ped/topic2005.htm> (27 April 2006).

Crook, J. et al. Interstitial brachytherapy for penile cancer: an alternative to amputation. J. Urol. 167 (2002): 506-511.

Crystal P. and Strano S. To the editor. New Engl. J. Med. 354 (2006): 765-767.

Cunningham, J.D. et al. Malignant small bowel neoplasms: histopathologic determinants of recurrence and survival. Ann. Surg. 225 (1997): 300-306.

Cuttler, J. Health benefits of low-dose radiation (LDR): the science and medical applications. RSH Newsletter. 1 April 2004.

Cuttler, J.M. and Pollycove, M. Can cancer be treated with low doses of radiation? J. Am. Physicians Surgeons 8 (2003): 108-111.

Czito, B. et al. Adjuvant radiotherapy with and without concurrent chemotherapy for locally advanced transitional cell carcinoma of the renal pelvis and ureter. J. Urol. 172 (2004): 1271-1275.

Dabaja, B.S. et al. Adenocarcinoma of the small bowel: presentation, prognostic factors, and outcome of 217 patients. Cancer 101 (2004): 518-526.

Daily News Central. 11 cousins foil hereditary stomach cancer. 20 June 2006 <http://health.dailynewscentral.com/content/view/0002311/37/>   7 July 2006.

Damber, L. et al. Thyroid cancer after X-ray treatment of benign disorders of the cervical spine in adults. Acta Oncol. 41 (2002): 25-28.

Danaei, G. et al. Causes of cancer in the world: comparative risk assessment of nine behavioural and environmental risk factors. Lancet 366 (2005): 1784-1793.

D'Antonio, J. Chronic myelogenous leukemia. Clin. J. Oncol. Nurs. 9 (2005): 535-538. See erratum in Clin. J. Oncol. Nurs. 9 (2005): 672.

Darzy, K.H. and Shalet, S.M. Radiation-induced growth hormone deficiency. Horm. Res. 59 (2003): 1-11.

de la Vega, F.A. et al. Hyperfractionated radiotherapy and concomitant cisplatin for locally advanced laryngeal and hypopharyngeal carcinomas: final results of a single institutional program. Am. J. Clin. Oncol. 26 (2003): 550-557.

de Vries, W.J. and Long, M.A. Treatment of mesothelioma in Bloemfontein, South Africa. Eur. J. Cardiothoracic. Surg. 24 (2003): 434-440.

Deegan, W.F. Emerging strategies for the treatment of retinoblastoma. Curr. Opin. Ophthalmol. 14 (2003): 291-295.

del Regato, J.A., Trailins, A.H. and Pittman, D.D. Twenty years follow-up of patients with inoperable cancer of the prostate (stage C) treated by radiotherapy: report of a national cooperative study. Int. J. Radiat. Oncol. Biol. Phys. 26 (1993): 197-201.

DeLaney, T.F. et al. Neoadjuvant chemotherapy and radiotherapy for Large extremity soft-tissue sarcomas. Int. J. Radiat. Oncol. Biol. Phys. 56 (2003): 1117-1127.

DeNavas-Walt, C., Proctor, B.D. and Lee, C.H. U.S. Census Bureau, current population reports, P60-229, income, poverty, and health insurance coverage in the United States: 2004. U.S. Government Printing Office, Washington DC, 2005.

Deniaud-Alexandre, E. et al. Results of definitive irradiation in a series of 305 epidermoid carcinomas of the anal canal. Int. J. Radiat. Oncol. Biol. Phys. 56 (2003): 1259-1273.

Denis, F. et al. Final results of the 94-01 French Head and Neck Oncology and Radiotherapy Group randomized trial comparing radiotherapy alone with concomitant radiochemotherapy in advanced-stage oronopharynx carcinoma. J. Clin. Oncol. 22 (2004): 69-76.

Derenzini, E. et al. Treatment of colorectal cancer liver metastases. Minerva Med. 97 (2006): 107-119.

DeVries, A. et al. The role of radiotherapy in the treatment of malignant meningiomas. Strahlenther. Onkol. 175 (1999): 62-67.

Devrup, A.T. and Weiss, S.W. Grading of soft tissue sarcomas: the challenge of providing precise information in an imprecise world. Histopathology 48 (2006): 42-50.

Dezube, B.J. Acquired immunodeficiency syndrome-related Kaposi's sarcoma: clinical features, staging, and treatment. Semin. Oncol. 27 (2000): 424-430.

Diehl, V. et al. Hodgkin's lymphoma: biology and treatment strategies for primary, refractory, and relapsed disease. Hematology 2003:225-247.

Diem, E. et al. Non-thermal DNA breakage by mobile-phone radiation (1800 MHz) in human fibroblasts and in transformed GFSH-R17 rat granulose cells in vitro. Mutat. Res. 583 (2005): 178-183.

Dillman, R.O. et al. A randomized trial of induction chemotherapy plus high-dose radiation versus radiation alone in stage III non-small-cell lung cancer. N. Engl. J. Med. 323 (1990): 940-945.

Dinney, C. Therapy of invasive bladder cancer, Urology. 67 (2006): 56-59.

Doll, R. and Wakeford, R. Risk of childhood cancer from fetal irradiation. Br. J. Radiol. 70 (1997): 130-139.

Dominick, K.L. et al. Provider characteristics and mammography recommendation among women in their 40s and 50s. J. Womens Health, 12 (2003): 61-71.

Dubois, J.B., Azria, D. and Ychou, M. External beam radiation therapy and interstitial brachytherapy in the treatment of anal canal carcinomas: a series of 70 patients. Bull. Cancer. 90 (2003): 1107-1110.

Duncan, W. et al. Carcinoma of the prostate: results of radical radiotherapy (1970-1985). Int. J. Radiat. Oncol. Biol. Phys. 26 (1993): 203-210.

Early Breast Cancer Trialists' Collaborative Group. Favourable and unfavourable effects on long-term survival of radiotherapy for early breast cancer: an overview of the randomised trials. Lancet 355 (2000): 1757-1770.

Eastman Kodak Co., interview by Ben Dobbin. Kodak develops faster, safer X-ray film. 9 March 2005. <http://news.yahoo.com/news?tmpl=story&u=/ap/20050309/ap_on_bige/safer_x_ray> (9 March 2005).

Eifel, P.J. et al. Pelvic irradiation with concurrent chemotherapy versus pelvic and para-aortic irradiation for high-risk cervical cancer: an update of radiation therapy oncology group trial (RTOG) 90-01. J. Clin. Oncol. 22 (2004): 872-880.

Einhorn, N. et al. A systematic overview of radiation therapy effects in ovarian cancer. Acta Oncol. 42 (2003): 562-566.

Eisbruch, A. et al. Recurrences near base of skull after IMRT for head-and-neck cancer: implications for target delineation in high neck and for parotid gland sparing. Int. J. Radiat. Oncol. Biol. Phys. 59 (2004): 28-42.

Eksteen, E.C. et al. Comparison of voice characteristics following three different methods of treatment for laryngeal cancer. J. Otolaryngol. 32 (2003): 250-253.

El-Deiry, W.S. Colon cancer, adenocarcinoma, updated 20 April 2006 <http://www.emedicine.com/med/topic413.htm> 8 July 2006.

Elekta, Inc. Gamma Knife® surgery reimbursement for 2006 solidifies efficacy of technology as standard of care in radiosurgery. 12 January 2006. <http://www.elekta.com/site_dbase.php?form_link_id=2593916> (19 June 2006).

Elmore, J.G. et al. Variability in radiologists' interpretations of mammograms. N. Engl. J. Med. 331 (1994):1493-1499.

Elmore, J.G. et al. The association between obesity and screening mammography accuracy. Arch. Intern. Med. 164 (2004): 1140-1147.

Emmanouilides, C. Radioimmunotherapy for Waldenstrom's macroglobulinemia. Semin. Oncol. 30 (2003): 258-261.

Eng, T.Y. et al. Treatment of merkel cell carcinoma. Am. J. Clin. Oncol. 27 (2004): 510-515.

Epstein, S.S. The politics of cancer revisited. Fremont Center: East Ridge Press, 1998.

Epstein, S.S., Bertell, R. and Seaman, B. Dangers and unreliability of mammography: breast examination is a safe, effective, and practical alternative. Int. J. Health Serv. 31 (2001): 605-615.

European Study Group for Pancreatic Cancer. A randomized trial of chemoradiotherapy and chemotherapy after resection of pancreatic cancer. N. Engl. J. Med. 350 (2004): 1200-1210.

Falkmer, U. et al. A systematic overview of radiation therapy effects in skeletal metastases. Acta Oncol. 42 (2003): 620-633.

Faria, P. et al. Focal versus diffuse anaplasia in Wilms tumor--new definitions with prognostic significance: a report from the National Wilms Tumor Study Group. Am. J. Surg. Pathol. 20 (1996): 909-920.

Feigenberg, S.J. et al. Angiosarcoma after breast-conserving therapy: experience with hyperfractionated radiotherapy. Int. J. Radiat. Oncol. Biol. Phys. 52 (2002): 620-626.

Ferrer, F. et al. Impact of radiotherapy on local control and survival in uterine sarcomas: a retrospective study from the Grup Oncologic Catala-Occita. Int. J. Radiat. Oncol. Biol. Phys. 44 (1999): 47-52.

Fesinmeyer, M.D. et al. Differences in survival by histologic type of pancreatic cancer. Cancer Epidemiol. Biomarkers Prev. 14 (2005): 1766-1773.

Finch, E. CTSI: full speed ahead, posted July 2002. <http://www.imagingeconomics.com/library/200207-09.asp> (9 June 2004).

Finger, P.T. Radiation therapy for choroidal melanoma. Surv. Ophthalmol. 42 (1997): 215-232.

Finger, P.T. et al. Palladium-103 plaque radiotherapy for choroidal melanoma: an 11-year study. Int. J. Radiat. Oncol. Biol. Phys. 54 (2002): 1438-1445.

Fink, C.A. and Bates, M.N. Melanoma and ionizing radiation: is there a causal relationship? Radiat. Res. 164 (2005): 701-710.

Firat, S., Murray, K. and Erickson, B. High-dose whole abdominal and pelvic irradiation for treatment of ovarian carcinoma: long-term toxicity and outcomes. Int. J. Radiat. Oncol. Biol., Phys. 57 (2003): 201-207.

Fisher, B. et al. Lumpectomy and radiation therapy for the treatment of intraductal breast cancer: findings from National Surgical Adjuvant Breast and Bowel Project B-17. J. Clin. Oncol. 16 (1998): 441-452.

Fisher B et al. Twenty-year follow-up of a randomized trial comparing total mastectomy, lumpectomy, and lumpectomy plus irradiation for the treatment of invasive breast cancer. N. Engl. J. Med. 347 (2002): 1233-1241.

Fitzgerald, R.C. and Caldas, C. Clinical implications of E-cadherin associated hereditary diffuse gastric cancer. Gut 53 (2004): 775-778.

Fletcher, S.W. Whither scientific deliberation in health policy recommendations? – Alice in the wonderland of breast cancer screening. N. Engl. J. Med. 336 (1997): 1180-1183.

Fong, Y. et al. An analysis of 412 cases of hepatocellular carcinoma at a Western center. Ann. Surg. 229 (1999): 790-799.

Foo, M.L. et al. External radiation therapy and transcatheter iridium in the treatment of extrahepatic bile duct carcinoma. Int. J. Radiat. Oncol. Biol. Phys. 39 (1997): 929-935.

Fontanesi, J. et al. Interstitial iodine 125 and concomitant cisplatin followed by hyperfractionated external beam irradiation for malignant supratentorial glioma. Preliminary experience at the University of Tennessee, Memphis. Am. J. Clin. Oncol. 16 (1993): 412-417.

Forastiere, A.A. et al. Concurrent chemotherapy and radiotherapy for organ preservation in advanced laryngeal cancer. N. Engl. J. Med. 349 (2003): 2091-2098.

Ford, D. et al. External beam radiotherapy in the management of differentiated thyroid cancer. Clin. Oncol. 15 (2003): 337-341.

Fortney, J.T. et al. Anesthesia for pediatric external beam radiation therapy. Int. J. Radiat. Oncol. Biol. Phys. 44 (1999): 587-591.

Fraker, D.L. Update on the management of parathyroid tumors. Curr. Opin. Oncol. 12 (2000): 41-48.

Franchin, G. et al. Radiotherapy for patients with early-stage glottic carcinoma: univariate and multivariate analyses in a group of consecutive, unselected patients. Cancer 98 (2003): 765-772.

Frank, S.J. et al. Definitive radiation therapy for squamous cell carcinoma of the vagina. Int. J. Radiat. Oncol. Biol. Phys. 62 (2005): 138-147.

Frigerio, L. et al. Adjunctive radiotherapy after radical hysterectomy in high risk early stage cervical carcinoma. Assessment of morbidity and recurrences. Eur. J. Gynaecol. Oncol. 15 (1994): 132-137.

Frustaci, S. et al. Adjuvant chemotherapy for adult soft tissue sarcomas of the extremeties and girdles: results of the Italian randomized cooperative trial. J. Clin. Oncol. 19 (2001): 1238-1247.

Fuchs, B. et al. Complications in long-term survivors of Ewing sarcoma. Cancer 98 (2003): 2687-2692.

Fury, M.G. et al. A 14-year retrospective review of angiosarcoma: clinical characteristics, prognostic factors, and treatment outcomes with surgery and chemotherapy. Cancer J. 11 (2005): 241-247. See erratum in Cancer J. 11 (2005): 354.

Gambus, G. et al. Prevalence and distribution of HHV-8 in different subpopulations, with and without HIV infection, in Spain, AIDS, 15 (2001): 1167-1174.

Garaventa, A. et al. Localized unresectable neuroblastoma: results of treatment based on clinical prognostic factors. Annal. Oncol. 13 (2002): 956-964.

Garcia, J.A. and Dreicer, R. Adjuvant and neoadjuvant chemotherapy for bladder cancer: management and controversies. Nat. Clin. Pract. Urol. 2 (2005): 32-37.

Gardner, B.G. et al. Normal tissue sequelae in the second decade after high dose radiation therapy with combined photons and conformal protons for locally advanced prostate cancer. J. Urol. 167 (2002): 123-126.

Garwicz, S. et al. Second malignant neoplasms after cancer in childhood and adolescence: a population-based case-control study in the 5 Nordic Countries. The Nordic Society for Pediatric Hematology and Oncology. The Association of the Nordic Cancer Registries. Int. J. Cancer 88 (2000): 672-678.

Gauden, S., Ramsay, J. and Tripcony, L. The curative treatment by radiotherapy alone of stage I non-small cell carcinoma of the lung. Chest 108 (1995): 1278-1282.

Gebski, V. et al. Survival effects of postmastectomy adjuvant radiation therapy using biologically equivalent doses: a clinical perspective. J. Natl. Cancer Inst. 98 (2006): 26-38.

Georg, D. et al. Impact of micromultileaf collimator on stereotactic radiotherapy of uveal melanoma. Int. J. Radiat. Oncol. Biol. Phys. 55 (2003): 881-891.

Gerecitano, J. and Straus, D.J. Treatment of Burkitt lymphoma in adults. Expert Rev. Anticancer Ther. 6 (2006): 373-381.

Gershenson, D.M. Update on malignant ovarian germ cell tumors. Cancer 71 (1993): 1581-1590.

Gerstle, J.T., Kauffman, G.L., Jr. and Koltun, W.A. The incidence, management, and outcome of patients with gastrointestinal carcinoids and secondary primary malignancies. J. Am. Coll. Surg. 180 (1995): 427-432.

Gerszten, K. et al. The impact of adjuvant radiotherapy on carcinosarcoma of the uterus. Gynecol. Oncol. 68 (1998): 8-13.

Gezairy, H.A. Regional consultation on lung cancer prevention and control. Cairo, Egypt. 21-23 June 2004. <http://www.emro.who.int/ncd/news-LungCancer0604 RDmessage.htm> (6 June 2006).

Ghosh, A.K., Lundstrom, C.E. and Edwards, W.D. Radiation arteritis following treatment for Wilms' tumor: an unusual case of weight loss. Vasc. Med. 7 (2002): 19-23.

Giordano, S.H., Buzdar, A.U. and Hortobagyi, G.N. Breast carcinoma in men. Ann. Intern. Med. 137 (2002): 678-687.

Giralt, S. et al. 166Ho-DOTMP plus melphalan followed by peripheral blood stem cell transplantation in patients with multiple myeloma: Results of two phase 1/2 Trials, Blood 102 (2003): 2684-2691.

Gofman, J.W. Radiation-induced cancer from low-dose exposure: an independent analysis. Committee Nuclear Responsibility, 1990.

Goh, L-A., Peh, W.C.G. and Shek, T.W.H. Giant cell tumor, updated 6 June 2002. <http://www.emedicine.com/radio/topic307.htm> (15 July 2006).

Gonzalez Gonzalez, D. et al. Role of radiotherapy, in particular intraluminal brachytherapy, in the treatment of proximal bile duct carcinoma. Ann. Oncol. 10 (1999): 215-220.

Gopal, A. and Budoff, M.J. Coronary calcium scanning. Am. Heart Hosp. J. 4 (2006): 43-50.

Gores, G.J. Early detection and treatment of cholangiocarcinoma. Liver Transpl. 6 (2000): S30-S34.

Gotzsche, P.C. and Olsen, O. Is screening for breast cancer with mammography justifiable? Lancet 355 (2000): 129-134.

Gowda, R.V. et al. Three weeks radiotherapy for T1 glottic cancer: the Christie and Royal Marsden Hospital experience. Radiother. Oncol. 68 (2003): 105-111.

Grabenbauer, G.G. et al. Interstitial brachytherapy with Ir-192 low-dose-rate in the treatment of primary and recurrent cancer of the oral cavity and oronopharynx. Review of 318 patients treated between 1985 and 1997. Strahlenther Onkol. 177 (2001): 338-344.

Graf, R. et al. Impact of overall treatment time on local control of anal cancer treated with radiochemotherapy. Oncology 65 (2003): 14-22.

Grau, J.J. et al. Impact of adjuvant therapy in the long-term outcome of patients with resected gastric cancer. J. Surg. Oncol. 82 (2003): 234-240.

Greenlee, R.T. et al. Cancer statistics, 2000. CA Cancer J. Clin. 50 (2000): 7-33.

Greenlee, R.T. et al. Cancer statistics, 2001. CA Cancer J. Clin. 50 (2000): 15-36. See erratum CA Cancer J. Clin. 51 (2001): 144.

Grégoire, V. and Maingon, P. Intensity-modulated radiation therapy in head and neck squamous cell carcinoma: an adaptation of 2-dimensional concepts or a reconsideration of current clinical practice. Sem. Radiat. Oncol. 14 (2004): 110-120.

Greisinger, A.J. et al. Terminally ill cancer patients: their most important concerns. Cancer Pract. 5 (1997): 147-154.

Grigsby, P.W. et al. Radiation therapy for carcinoma of the cervix with biopsy-proven positive para-aortic lymph nodes. Int. J. Radiat. Oncol. Biol. Phys. 49 (2001): 733-738.

Grossman, H.B. et al. Surveillance for recurrent bladder cancer using a point-of-care proteomic assay. J. Am. Med. Assoc. 295 (2006): 299-305.

Guerrero Urbano, M.T. and Nutting, C.M. Clinical use of intensity-modulated radiotherapy: part II. Br. J. Radiol. 77 (2004): 177-182.

Gustavsson, A., Osterman, B. and Cavallin-Stahl, E. A systematic overview of radiation therapy effects in Hodgkin's lymphoma. Acta Oncol. 42 (2003): 589-604.

Haas, R.L. et al. Response rates and lasting remissions after low-dose involved field radiotherapy in indolent lymphomas. J. Clin. Oncol. 21 (2003): 2474-2480.

Haas-Kogan, D.A. et al. Impact of radiotherapy for high-risk neuroblastoma: a children's cancer group study. Int. J. Radiat. Oncol. Biol. Phys. 56 (2003): 28-39.

Habrand, J.L. et al. The role of radiation therapy in the management of craniopharyngioma: a 25-year experience and review of the literature. Int. J. Radiat. Oncol. Biol. Phys. 44 (1999): 255-263.

Hacker, N.F. Current management of early vulvar cancer. Ann. Acad. Med. Singapore 27 (1998): 688-692.

Hall, E.J. and Wuu, C.S. Radiation-induced second cancers: the impact of 3D-CRT and IMRT. Int. J. Radiat. Oncol. Biol. Phys. 56 (2003): 83-88.

Hamilton, A.S. et al. Health outcomes after external-beam radiation therapy for clinically localized prostate cancer: results from the Prostate Cancer Outcomes Study. J. Clin. Oncol. 19 (2001): 2517-2526.

Hanabusa, K. et al. Acoustic neuroma with malignant transformation. J. Neurosurg. 95 (2001): 518-521.

Han, M. et al. Long-term biochemical disease-free and cancer-specific survival following anatomic radical retropubic prostatectomy. Urol. Clin. North Am. 28 (2001): 555-565.

Hanlon, A.L. et al. Chronic rectal bleeding after high-dose conformal treatment of prostate cancer warrants modification of existing morbidity scales. Int. J. Radiat. Oncol. Biol. Phys. 38 (1997): 59-63.

Hardell, L., Carlberg, M. and Mild, K.H. Case-control study of the association between the use of cellular and cordless telephones and malignant brain tumors diagnosed during 2000-2003. Environ. Res. 100 (2006): 232-241.

Hartmann, J.T. et al. Prognostic variables for response and outcome in patients with extragonadal germ-cell tumors. Ann. Oncol. 13 (2002): 1017-1028.

Harvey, B.J. et al. Effect of breast self-examination techniques on the risk of death from breast cancer. Can. Med. Assoc. J. 157 (1997): 1205-1212.

Haselkorn, T., Whittemore, A.S. and Lilienfeld, D.E. Incidence of small bowel cancer in the United States and worldwide: geographic, temporal, and racial differences. Cancer Causes Control. 16 (2005): 781-787.

Hashim, A.R. and Al-Quryni, A.M. Carcinoma of unknown primary site. Saudi Med. J. 26 (2005): 47-50.

Haupt, R. et al. Epidemiological aspects of craniopharyngioma. J. Pediatr. Endocrinol. Metab. 19 (2006): 289-93.

Hazard, L., O'Connor, J. and Scaife, C. Role of radiation therapy in gastric adenocarcinoma. 12 (2006): 1511-1520.

Health Daily News Central. Hodgkin's specialists to review Texas teen's case, posted September 7, 2005. <http://health.dailynewscentral.com/index2.php?option=content&task> (April 28, 2006).

Health Physics Society. Radiation risk in perspective, revised August 2004. <http://www.hps.org/documents/radiationrisk.pdf> (31 May 2006).

Heeg et al. In vitro transformation models: modeling human cancer. Cell Cycle 5 (2006): 630-634.

Heidenreich, P.A. et al. Asymptomatic cardiac disease following mediastinal irradiation. J. Am. Coll. Cardiol. 42 (2003): 743-749.

Hempelmann, L.H. et al. Neoplasms in persons treated with X-rays in infancy: fourth survey in 20 years. J. Natl. Cancer Inst. 55 (1975): 519-530.

Hennig, R., Ding, X.Z. and Adrian, T.E. On the role of the islets of Langerhans in pancreatic cancer. Histol. Histopathol. 19 (2004): 999-1011.

Hensley, M.L. Uterine/female genital sarcomas. Curr. Treat. Options Oncol. 1 (2000): 161-168.

Hentschel, S.J. and McCutcheon, I.E. Stereotactic radiosurgery for Cushing disease. Neurosurg. Focus 16 (2004): E5.

Herfarth, K.K. et al. Stereotactic single-dose radiation therapy of liver tumors: results of a phase I/II trial. J. Clin. Oncol. 19 (2001): 164-170.

Herman, J.M. et al. Repeat gamma knife radiosurgery for refractory or recurrent trigeminal neuralgia: treatment outcomes and quality-of-

Life assessment. Int. J. Radiat. Oncol. Biol. Phys. 59 (2004): 112-116.

Herwig, R. et al. Late urologic effects after adjuvant irradiation in stage I endometrial carcinoma. Urol. 63 (2004): 354-358.

Hodgson, D.C. et al. Evolution of treatment for Hodgkin's disease: a population-based study of radiation therapy use and outcome. Clin. Oncol. 15 (2003): 255-263.

Hofmann, W.K. et al. Myelodysplastic syndromes. Hematol. J. 5 (2004): 1-8.

Hollister, L.E. Health aspects of cannabis: revisited. Int. J. Neuropsychopharmacol. 1 (1998): 71-80.

Holy Name Hospital, interview by Varian Medical Systems. Varian Medical Systems and GE Healthcare collaboration enables pioneering radiotherapy treatment. 20 October 2004. <http://varian.mediaroom.com/index.php?s=home&item=145&printable> (21 April 2006).

Holzbeierlein, J.M., Sogani, P.C. and Sheinfeld, J. Histology and clinical outcomes in patients with bilateral testicular germ cell tumors: the Memorial Sloan Kettering Cancer Center experience 1950 to 2001. J. Urol. 169 (2003): 2122-2125.

Homs, M.Y. et al. Predictors of outcome of single-dose brachytherapy for the palliation of dysphagia from esophageal cancer. Brachytherapy. 1 (2006): 41-48.

Hong, T.S., et al. Intensity-modulated radiation therapy: emerging cancer treatment technology. Br. J. Cancer. 92 (2005): 1819-1824.

Horwich, A. and Swerdlow, A.J. Second primary breast cancer after Hodgkin's disease. Br. J. Cancer 90 (2004): 294-298.

Hoskin, P.J. Bisphosphonates and radiation therapy for palliation of metastatic bone disease. Cancer Treat. Rev. 29 (2003): 321-327.

Hoybye, C. et al. Transsphenoidal surgery in Cushing Disease: 10 years of experience in 34 consecutive cases. J. Neurosurg. 100 (2004): 634-638.

Hoyert, D.L. and Anderson, R.N. Age-adjusted death rates: trend data based on the year 2000 standard population. Natl. Vital Stat. Rep. 49 (2001): 1-8.

Hu, D.N. et al. Population-based incidence of uveal melanoma in various races and ethnic groups. Am. J. Ophthalmol. 140 (2005): 612-617.

Huff, J.S. Neoplasms, brain, updated 22 March 2005. <http://www.emedicine.com/emerg/topic334.htm> (6 June 2006).

Hujoel, P.P. et al. Antepartum dental radiography and infant low birth weight. J. Am. Med. Assoc. 291 (2004): 1987-1993.

Hull, G.W. et al. Cancer control with radical prostatectomy alone in 1,000 consecutive patients. J. Urol. 167 (2002): 528-534.

Hurria, A. and Kris, M.G. Management of lung cancer in older adults. Cancer J. Clinicians 53 (2003): 325-341.

Irvin, W.P., Rice, L.W. and Berkowitz, R.S. Advances in the management of endometrial adenocarcinoma. A review. J. Repro. Med. 47 (2002): 173-189.

Ito, H. et al. Treatment outcomes associated with surgery for gallbladder cancer: a 20-year experience. J. Gastrointest. Surg. 8 (2004): 183-190.

Ivanov, V.K. et al. Thyroid cancer among "liquidators" of the Chernobyl accident. Br. J. Radiol. 70 (1997): 937-941.

Ivanov, V.K. et al. Radiation-epidemiological studies of thyroid cancer incidence among children and adolescents in the Bryansk oblast of Russia after the Chernobyl accident (1991-2001 follow-up period). Radiat. Environ. Biophys. (2006):

Janda, M. et al. Impaired quality of life in patients commencing radiotherapy for cancer. Strahlenther. Onkol. 180 (2004): 78-83.

Jani, A.B., Roeske, J.C. and Rash, C. Intensity-modulated radiation therapy for prostate cancer. Clin. Prostate Cancer 2 (2003): 98-105.

Jasmin, L.D. Hypothalamic tumor, updated 16 November 2004. <http://www.nlm.nih.gov/medlineplus/ency/article/001211.htm> (6 June 2006).

Jawahar, A. et al. Management strategies for patients with brain metastases: has radiosurgery made a difference? South Med. J. 97 (2004): 254-258.

Jazieh, A.R. and Buncher, C.R. Racial and age-related disparities in obtaining screening mammography: results of a statewide database. South Med. J. 95 (2002): 1145-1148.

Jemal, A. et al. Cancer statistics, 2002. CA Cancer J. Clin. 52 (2002): 23-47. See erratum CA Cancer J. Clin. 52 (2002): 119, 181-182.

Jemal, A. et al. Cancer statistics, 2003. CA Cancer J. Clin. 53 (2003): 5-26.

Jemal, A. et al. Cancer statistics, 2004. CA Cancer J. Clin. 54 (2004): 8-29

Jemal, A. et al. Cancer statistics, 2005. CA Cancer J. Clin. 55 (2005): 10-30. See erratum CA Cancer J. Clin. 55 (2005): 259.

Jemal, A. et al. Cancer statistics, 2006. CA Cancer J. Clin. 56 (2006): 106-130.

Jennings, R.W. et al. Fetal neuroblastoma: prenatal diagnosis and natural history. J. Pediatr. Surg. 28 (1993): 1168-1174.

Jereczek-Fossa, B.A. Postoperative irradiation in endometrial cancer: still a matter of controversy. Cancer Treat. Rev. 27 (2001): 19-33.

Jereczek-Fossa, B.A. et al. Radiotherapy-induced thyroid disorders. Cancer Treat. Rev. 30 (2004): 369-384.

Johansson, J.E. et al. Fifteen-year survival in prostate cancer. A prospective, population-based study in Sweden. J. Am. Med. Assoc. 277 (1997): 467-471.

Johns Hopkins Pancreas Cancer Web. National familial pancreas tumor registry, posted 13 November 2005. <http://pathology2.jhu.edu/pancreas/nfptr.cfm> (7 June 2006).

Johnson, S.R. et al. A single center experience with extrahepatic cholangiocarcinomas. Surgery 130 (2001): 584-590.

Johnston, J.B. et al. Long-term outcome following treatment of hairy cell leukemia with pentostatin (nipent): a National Cancer Institute of Canada Study. Semin. Oncol. 27 (2000): 32-36.

Jones, R.H. and Vasey, P.A. Part I: testicular cancer—management of early disease. Lancet Oncol. 4 (2003): 730-737.

Jönsson, H. and Mattson, S. Excess radiation absorbed doses from non-optimised radioiodine treatment of hyperthyroidism. Radiat. Protect. Dos. 108 (2004): 107-114.

Kachnic, J. et al. Bladder preservation by combined modality therapy for invasive bladder cancer. Clin. Oncol. 15 (1997): 1022-1029.

Kaiser, C.P. Pioneering CT screening centers close doors. 11 February 2003. <http://www.diagnosticimaging.com/dinews/2003021101.shtml> (11 February 2003).

Kaneko, S. et al. Trend of brain tumor incidence by histological subtypes in Japan: estimation from the Brain Tumor Registry of Japan, 1973-1993. J. Neuro-Oncol. 60 (2002): 61-69.

Kapiteijn, E. et al. Preoperative radiotherapy combined with total mesorectal excision for resectable rectal cancer. N. Engl. J. Med. 345 (2001): 638-646.

Karim, A.B. et al. Randomized trial on the efficacy of radiotherapy for cerebral low-grade glioma in the adult: European Organization for Research and Treatment of Cancer Study 22845 with the Medical Research Council study BRO4: an interim analysis. Int. J. Radiat. Oncol. Biol. Phys. 52 (2002): 316-324.

Kasamon, Y. and Swinnen, L.J. Treatment advances in Burkitt lymphoma and leukemia. Curr. Opinion Oncol. 16 (2004): 429-435.

Katz, A. et al. The role of radiation therapy in preventing regional recurrences of invasive squamous cell carcinoma of the vulva. Int. J. Radiat. Oncol. Biol. Phys. 57 (2003): 409-418.

Kaurah, P. and Huntsman, D.G. Hereditary diffuse gastric cancer, updated 13 December 2004. <http://www.geneclinics.org/profiles/hgc/index.html> (11 July 2006).

Kerlikowske, K. et al. Variability and accuracy in mammographic interpretation using the American College of Radiology breast imaging reporting and data system. J. Natl. Cancer Inst. 90 (1998): 1801-1809.

Kerlikowske, K., et al. Performance of screening mammography among women with and without a first-degree relative with breast cancer. Ann. Intern. Med. 133 (2000): 855-863.

Keys, H.M. et al. A phase III trial of surgery with or without adjunctive external pelvic radiation therapy in intermediate risk endometrial adenocarcinoma: a gynecologic oncology group study. Gynecol. Oncol. 92 (2004): 744-751.

Khan, D.C. et al. Radiotherapy for the treatment of giant cell tumor of the spine: a report of six cases and review of the literature. Cancer Invest. 17 (1999): 110-113.

Khoury, J.D. Ewing sarcoma family of tumors. Adv. Anat. Pathol. 12 (2005): 212-220.

Kim, S. et al. Role of postoperative radiotherapy in the management of extrahepatic bile duct cancer. Int. J. Radiat. Oncol. Biol. Phys. 54 (2002): 414-419.

Kim, S. et al. Predicting outcome and directing therapy for papillary thyroid carcinoma. Arch. Surg. 139 (2004): 390-394.

Kimura, Y. et al. Stage I and II mobile tongue carcinomas treated by external radiation and gold seed implantation. Acta Oncol. 42 (2003): 763-770.

Kirkbride, P. et al. Outcome of curative management of malignant tumours of the parotid gland. J. Otolaryngol. 30 (2001): 271-279.

Kirkwood, J.M. et al. Interferon alfa-2b adjuvant Therapy of High-Risk resected cutaneous melanoma: the Eastern Cooperative Oncology Group Trial EST 1684. J. Clin. Oncol. 14 (1996): 7-17.

Kleinberg, L. et al. Mature survival results with preoperative cisplatin, protracted infusion 5 fluorouracil, and 44-Gy radiotherapy for esophageal cancer. Int. J. Radiat. Oncol. Biol. Phys. 56 (2003): 328-334.

Knocke, T.H. et al. Results of postoperative radiotherapy in the treatment of sarcoma of the corpus uteri. Cancer 83 (1998): 1972-1979.

Kodera, Y. et al. Chemotherapy as a component of multimodal therapy for gastric carcinoma. World J. Gastroenterol. 12 (2006): 2000-2005.

Kollmorgen, C.F. et al. The long-term effect of adjuvant postoperative chemoradiotherapy for rectal carcinoma on bowel function. Ann. Surg. 220 (1994): 676-682.

Konstantakos, A.K. and Dudgeon, D.L. Liposarcoma, updated 19 August 2002. http://www.emedicine.com/PED/topic1317.htm> (27 April 2006).

Konstantakos, A.K. and Graham, D.J. Thyroid, anaplastic carcinoma, updated 18 April 2006. <http://www.emedicine.com/MED/topic2687.htm> (7 June 2006).

Kopans, D.B., Halpern, E. and Hulka, C.A. Statistical power in breast cancer screening trials and mortality reduction among women 40-49 years of age with particular emphasis on the National Breast Screening Study of Canada. Cancer 74 (1994): 1196-1203.

Koschker, A.C. et al. 2006. Adrenocorticol carcinoma–improving patient care by establishing new structures. Exp. Clin. Endocrinol. Diabetes 114:45-51.

Koshy, M. et al. Radiation-induced osteosarcomas in the pediatric population. Int. J. Radiat. Oncol. Biol. Phys. 63 (2005): 1169-1174.

Kovacs, A.F. et al. Postoperative chemotherapy with cisplatin and 5-flurorouracil in cancer of the oral cavity and the oropharynx—long-term results. J. Chemother. 15 (2003): 495-502.

Kovacs, A.F. Intra-arterial induction high-dose chemotherapy with cisplatin for oral and oropharyngeal cancer: long-term results. Br. J. Cancer 90 (2004): 1323-1328.

Kricker, A. and Armstrong, B. Does sunlight have a beneficial influence on certain cancers? Prog. Biophys. Mol. Biol. 92 (2006): 132-139.

Krook, J.E. et al. Effective surgical adjuvant therapy for high-risk rectal carcinoma. N. Engl. J. Med. 324 (1991): 709-715.

Krzyzanowska, M.K. and Tannock, I.F. Should screen detected breast cancers be managed differently? J. Nat. Cancer Inst. 97 (2005): 1170-1171.

Kucera, H. et al. Radiotherapy alone for invasive vaginal cancer: outcome with intracavitary high dose rate brachytherapy versus conventional low dose rate brachytherapy. Acta Obstet. Gynecol. Scand. 80 (2001): 355-360.

Kujala, E., Makatie, T. and Kivela, T. Very long-term prognosis of patients with malignant uveal melanoma. Invest. Opththalmol. Vis. Sci. 44 (2003): 4651-4659.

Kumar, A. et al. Management of multiple myeloma: a systematic review and critical appraisal of published studies. Lancet Oncol. 4 (2003): 293-304.

Kupelian, P.A. et al. Radical prostatectomy, external beam radiotherapy <72 Gy, external beam radiotherapy > or =72 Gy, permanent seeds/external beam radiotherapy for stage T1-T2 prostate cancer. Int. J. Radiat. Oncol. Biol. Phys. 58 (2004): 25-33.

Kurzrock, R. Myelodysplastic syndrome overview. Semin. Hematol. 39 (2002): 18-25.

Kushner, D.M. et al. High dose rate ^{192}Ir afterloading brachytherapy for cancer of the vagina. Br. J. Radiol. 76 (2003): 719-725.

La Quaglia, M.P. et al. The impact of gross total resection on local control and survival in high-risk neuroblastoma. J. Pediatr. Surg. 39 (2004): 412-417.

Landoni, F. et al. Randomised study of radical surgery versus radiotherapy for stage Ib-IIa cervical cancer. Lancet 350 (1997): 535-540.

Lapeyre, M. et al. Postoperative brachytherapy alone and combined postoperative radiotherapy and brachytherapy boost for squamous cell carcinoma of the oral cavity, with positive or close margins. Head Neck 26 (2004): 216-223.

Lara, P.N., Jr. Malignant thymoma: current status and future directions, Cancer Treat. Rev. 26 (2000): 127-131.

Laukkanen, E. et al. The role of prophylactic brain irradiation in limited stage small cell lung cancer: clinical, neuropsychologic, and CT sequelae. Int. J. Radiat. Oncol. Biol. Phys. 14 (1988): 1109-1117.

Le Chevalier, T. et al. Radiotherapy alone versus combined chemotherapy and radiotherapy in nonresectable non-small-cell lung cancer: first analysis of a randomized trial in 353 patients. J. Natl. Cancer Inst. 83 (1991): 417-423.

le Maignan, C. et al. Three cycles of adriamycin, bleomycin, vinblastine, and dacarbazine (ABVD) or epirubicin, bleomycin, vinblastine, and methotrexate (EBVM) plus extended field radiation therapy in early and intermediate Hodgkin disease: 10-year results of a randomized trial. Blood 103 (2004): 58-66.

Leber, A.W. et al. Non-invasive intravenous coronary angiography using electron beam tomography and multislice computed tomography. Heart 89 (2003): 633-639.

Lee, S.J. et al. Initial therapy for chronic leukemia: playing the odds. J. Clinical Oncol. 16 (1998): 2897-2903.

Leitzmann, M. F. et al. Ejaculation frequency and subsequent risk of prostate cancer. J. Am. Med. Assoc. 291 (2004): 1578-1586.

Leone, N. et al. Surgery for carcinoma of the gallbladder. Our experience. Panminerva Med. 44 (2002): 227-231.

Leukaemia Research. Lymphatic cancer alliance, posted 2005. <http://www.lrf.org.uk/en/1/dislymhome.html> (20 June 2006).

Levine, S.C. Acoustic Neuroma-the basic facts, updated 16 December 1999. <http://www.med.umn.edu/otol/library/aneuroma/origin.htm> (1 June 2006).

Lewis, C. Full-body CT scans: what you need to know. FDA Consumer Magazine, November-December 2001.

Lim, A.J. et al. Quality of life: radical prostatectomy versus radiation therapy for prostate cancer. J. Urol. 154 (1995): 1420-1425.

Lin, J.C. et al. Phase III study of concurrent chemoradiotherapy versus radiotherapy alone for advanced nasopharyngeal carcinoma: positive effect on overall and progression-free survival. J. Clin. Oncol. 21 (2003): 631-637.

Liu, A.L., Wang, C.C. and Dai, K. Gamma knife radiosurgery for cavernous malformations, Zhongguo Yi Xue Ke Xue Yuan Xue Bao. 27 (2005): 18-21.

Liu, M.T. et al. Prognostic factors affecting the outcome of nasopharyngeal carcinoma. Jpn. J. Clin. Oncol. 33 (2003): 501-508.

Loeffler, J.S. et al. Radiosurgery as part of the initial management of patients with malignant gliomas. J. Clin. Oncol. 10 (1992): 1379-1385.

Lopes, M. Beatriz S. and Laws, E.R., Jr. Low-grade central nervous system tumors. Neurosurg. Focus 12 (2002): 1-7.

Longhi, A. et al. Height as a risk factor for osteosarcoma. J. Pediatr. Hematolo. Oncol. 27 (2005): 314-318.

Luckey, T.D. Radiation hormesis. CRC Press, 1991.

Lundkvist, et al. Proton therapy of cancer: potential clinical advantages and cost-effectiveness. Acta Oncol. 44 (2005): 850-861.

Mac Manus, M.P. and Hoppe, R.T. Is radiotherapy curative for stage I and II low-grade follicular lymphoma? Results of a long-term follow-up study of patients treated at Stanford University. J. Clin. Oncol. 14 (1996): 1282-1290.

Macdonald, D.R. Temozolomide for recurrent high-grade glioma, Seminars in Oncology 28 (2001): 3-12.

MacDonald, J.S. et al. Chemoradiotherapy after surgery compared with surgery alone for adenocarcinoma of the stomach or gastroesophageal junction. N. Engl. J. Med. 345 (2001): 725-730.

MacDonald, J.S. Adjuvant therapy for gastric cancer. Semin. Oncol. 30 (2003): 19-25.

MacEneaney, P.M. and Dachman, A.H. CT angiography review. Appl. Radiol. 29 (2000): 24-29.

Macieira-Coelho, A. Neoplastic disease through the human life span. Biogerontology 2 (2001): 179-192.

Maduro, J.H. et al. Acute and long-term toxicity following radiotherapy alone or in combination with chemotherapy for locally advanced cervical cancer. Cancer Treat. Rev. 29 (2003): 471-488.

Makary, M.A., et al. Multimodality treatment for esophageal cancer: the role of surgery and neoadjuvant therapy. Am. Surg. 69 (2003): 693-700.

Mackay, J. et al. The cancer atlas. American Cancer Society. Atlanta, Georgia, 2006.

Mancuso, A. and Sternberg, C.N. New treatments for metastatic kidney cancer. Can. J. Urol. 12 Suppl. 1 (2005): 66-70.

Marchese-Ragona, R., Marioni, G. and Staffieri, A. The unfinished *Turandot* and Puccini's laryngeal cancer. Laryngoscope 114 (2004): 911-914.

Martin, R.C. and Miller, J.H. Applications of californium-252 neutron sources in medicine, research and industry. Americas Nuclear Energy Symposium, 2002 Proceedings. 16-18 October 2002.

Martino, D. and Pass, H.I. Integration of multimodality approaches in the management of malignant pleural mesothelioma. Clin. Lung Cancer 5 (2004): 290-298.

Martling, A. et al. The Stockholm II trial on preoperative radiotherapy in rectal carcinoma: long-term follow-up of a population-based study. Cancer 92 (2001): 896-902.

Maruyama, Y. et al. A review of californium-252 neutron brachytherapy for cervical cancer. Cancer 68 (1991): 1189-1197.

Maruyama, Y. et al. Schedule in Cf-252 neutron brachytherapy: complications after delayed implant therapy for cervical cancer in phase II trial. Am. J. Clin. Oncol. 16 (1993): 168-174.

Mayer, R. et al. Hyperbaric oxygen and radiotherapy. Strahlenther Onkol. 181 (2005): 113-123.

McCaffrey, T.V. Thyroid cancer in the new millennium. Cancer Control 7 (2000): 209-210.

McIver, J.I. and Pollock, B.E. Radiation-induced tumor after stereotactic radiosurgery and whole brain radiotherapy: case report and literature review. J. Neurooncol. 66 (2004): 301-305.

McTiernan, A. Recent controversies in mammography screening for breast cancer, posted 19 April 2002. <http://www.medscape.com/viewarticle/430076> (28 May 2006).

Meier, S. et al. Survival and prognostic factors in patients with brain metastases from malignant melanoma. Onkologie 27 (2004): 145-149.

Meissner, H.I., Breen, N. and Yabroff, K.R. Whatever happened to clinical breast examinations? Am. J. Prev. Med. 25 (2003): 259-263.

Mell, L.K., Roeske, J.C. and Mundt, A.J. A survey of intensity-modulated radiation therapy use in the United States. Cancer 98 (2003): 204-211.

Mendenhall, W.M. et al. Giant cell tumor of bone. Am. J. Clin. Oncol. 29 (2006): 96-99.

Menvielle, G. et al. Smoking, alcohol drinking and cancer risk for various sites of the larynx and hypopharynx. A case control study in France. 13 (2004): 165-172.

Mettler, F.A., Jr. et al. CT scanning: patterns of use and dose. J. Radiol. Prot. 20 (2000): 353-359.

Meyer, T.A. et al. Small acoustic neuromas: surgical outcomes versus observation or radiation. Otol. Neurotol. 27 (2006): 380-392.

Meyerhardt, J.A. and Fuchs, C.S. Adjuvant therapy in gastric cancer: can we prevent recurrences? Oncology (Huntingt.) 17 (2003): 714-721.

Michell, M.J. and Al-Attar, M.A. Detection of subtle mammographic signs of malignancy. Appl. Radiol. 32 (2003): 11-16.

Micke, O. et al. Results and follow-up of locally advanced cancer of the exocrine pancreas treated with radiochemotherapy. Anticancer Res. 25 (2005): 1523-1530.

Miller, A.B. Is mammography screening for breast cancer really not justifiable? Recent Results Cancer Res. 163 (2003): 115-128.

Miller, T.P. Chemotherapy alone compared with chemotherapy plus radiotherapy for localized intermediate- and high-grade non-Hodgkin's Lymphoma. N. Engl. J. Med. 339 (1998): 21-26.

Milpied, N. et al. Initial treatment of aggressive lymphoma with high-dose chemotherapy and autologous stem-cell support. N. Engl. J. Med. 350 (2004): 1287-1295.

Minsky, B.D. et al. INT 0123 (Radiation Therapy Oncology Group 94-05) phase III trial of combined-modality therapy for esophageal cancer: high-dose versus standard-dose radiation therapy. J. Clin. Oncol. 20 (2002): 1167-1174.

Modlin, I.M., Lye, K.D. and Kidd, M. A 5-decade analysis of 13,715 carcinoid tumors. Cancer. 97 (2003): 934-959.

Modlin, I.M. et al. Current status of gastrointestinal carcinoids. Gastroenterology. 6 (2005): 1717-1751.

Moertel, C.G. Therapy of locally unresectable pancreatic carcinoma: a randomized comparison of high dose (600 rads) radiation alone, moderate dose radiation (4000 rads + 5-fluorouracil), and high dose radiation + 5-fluorouracil: The Gastrointestinal Tumor Study Group. Cancer 48 (1981): 1705-1710.

Mokbel, K. et al. Women's views on the introduction of annual screening mammography to those aged 40-49 years (a pilot study). Curr. Med. Res. Opin. 17 (2001): 111-112.

Mondragon-Sanchez, R. et al. A retrospective analysis of patients with gallbladder cancer treated with radical resection versus cholecystectomy plus external radiotherapy. Hepatogastroenterology 50 (2003): 1806-1810.

Monroe, A.T., Feigenberg, S.J. and Mendenhall, N.P. Angiosarcoma after breast-conserving therapy. Cancer 8 (2003): 132-1840.

Moss, E.L. et al. Toxicity, recurrence and survival after adjuvant radiotherapy treatment for FIGO stage I cancer of the endometrium. Clin. Oncol. 15 (2003): 250-254.

Mulford, D.A. and Jurcic, J.G. Antibody-based treatment of acute myeloid leukaemia. Expert Opin. Biol. Ther. 4 (2004): 95-105.

Muller, A.M. et al. Epidemiology of non-Hodgkin's lymphoma (NHL): trends, geographic distribution, and etiology. Ann. Hematol. 84 (2005): 1-12.

Multani, P., White, C.A. and Grillo-Lopez, A. Non-Hodgkin's lymphoma: review of conventional treatments. Curr. Pharm. Biotechnol. 2 (2001): 279-291.

Munson, N.D. et al. Parathyroid carcinoma: is there a role for adjuvant radiation therapy? Cancer 98 (2003): 2378-2384.

Nag, S. et al. Long-term follow-up of patients of intrahepatic malignancies treated with iodine-125 brachytherapy. Int. J. Radiat. Oncol. Biol. Phys. 64 (2006): 736-744.

Nakamura, K. et al. Multi-institutional analysis of early squamous cell carcinoma of the hypopharynx treated with radical radiotherapy. Int. J. Radiat. Oncol. Biol. Phys. 65 (2006): 1045-1050.

Nasti, G. et al. Impact of highly active antiretroviral therapy on the presenting features and outcome of patients with acquired immunodeficiency syndrome-related Kaposi sarcoma. Cancer 98 (2003): 2440-2446.

Nathan, P.C. et al. CNS-directed therapy in young children with T-lineage acute lymphoblastic leukemia: high-dose methotrexate versus cranial irradiation. Pediatr. Blood Cancer 42 (2004): 24-29.

National Academy of Sciences. Health risks from exposure to low levels of ionizing radiation. BEIR VII Phase 2. The National Academic Press, Washington, D.C., 2006.

National Association for Proton Therapy. Updated proton news, posted 23 February 2004. <http://www.proton-therapy.org/> (1 June 2006).

National Cancer Center. Cancer statistics in Japan 2005, posted 22 December 2005. <http://www.ncc.go.jp/en/statistics/2005/index.html> (25 February 2006).

National Cancer Institute. Radiation risks and pediatric computed tomography (CT): a guide for health care providers, posted 20 August 2002.

<http://www.cancer.gov/cancertopics/causes/radiation-risks-pediatric-CT> (10 June 2004).

National Cancer Institute. Merkel cell cancer fact sheet, reviewed 3 April 2003a. <http://www.cancer.gov/cancertopics/factsheet/Sites-Types/merkel-cell> (1 June 2006).

National Cancer Institute. The prostate cancer outcomes study: fact sheet, updated 2 May 2003b. <http://www.cancer.gov/newscenter/pcos> (30 March 2004).

National Cancer Institute, interview by Claudia Dreifus. A hopeful outlook on taming cancer. AARP Bulletin, December 2003.

National Cancer Institute. Cancer of unknown primary origin, reviewed 22 January 2004. <http://www.cancer.gov/cancertopics/factsheet/Sites-Types/unknownprimary> (28 April 2006).

National Cancer Institute. Testicular cancer: questions and answers, reviewed 24 May 2005a. <http://www.cancer.gov/cancertopics/factsheet/Sites-Types/testicular> (2 June 2006).

National Cancer Institute. General information about breast cancer, modified 22 June 2005b. <http://www.cancer.gov/cancertopics/pdq/treatment/breast> (6 June 2006).

National Cancer Institute. Waldenström's macroglobulinemia: questions and answers, reviewed 13 July 2005c. <http://www.cancer.gov/cancertopics/factsheet/Sites-Types/WM> (1 June 2006).

National Cancer Institute. Snapshots, revised August 2005d. <http://planning.cancer.gov/disease/snapshots.shtml> (31 May 2006).

National Cancer Institute. Carcinoma of unknown primary (PDQ®): treatment, modified 20 September 2005e. <http://www.cancer.gov/cancertopics/pdq/treatment/unknownprimary/HealthProfessional> (21 June 2006).

National Cancer Institute. Thymoma and thymic carcinoma (PDQ®): treatment, modified 30 September 2005f. <http://www.cancer.gov/cancertopics/pdq/treatment/malignant-thymoma/HealthProfessional> (30 June 2006).

National Cancer Institute. Surveillance, epidemiology, and end results (SEER) program (www.seer.cancer.gov) SEER*Stat Database: mortality - all COD, total U.S. (1969-2003) - linked to county attributes - Total U.S., 1969-2003 Counties, National Cancer Institute, DCCPS, Surveillance Research Program, Cancer

Statistics Branch, released January 2006a. Underlying mortality data provided by NCHS (www.cdc.gov/nchs).

National Cancer Institute. Small cell lung cancer (PDQ®): treatment, modified 6 March 2006b. <http://www.cancer.gov/cancertopics/pdq/treatment/small-cell-lung/healthprofessional/> (6 June 2006).

National Cancer Institute. Uterine sarcoma (PDQ®): treatment, modified 5 April 2006c. <http://www.cancer.gov/cancertopics/pdq/treatment/uterinesarcoma/healthprofessional> (2 June 2006).

National Cancer Institute. Genetics of medullary thyroid cancer (PDQ®), modified 1 May 2006d. <http://www.cancer.gov/cancertopics/pdq/genetics/medullarythyroid/healthprofessional> (7 June 2006).

National Cancer Institute. Ewing's family of tumors (PDQ®); treatment, modified 22 June 2006e <http://www.cancer.gov/cancertopics/pdq/treatment/ewings/HealthProfessional> (7 June 2006).

National Cancer Institute. Breast cancer surveillance consortium, no date. <http://breastscreening.cancer.gov/statistics/index.html> (2 May 2006).

National Institute of Diabetes and Digestive and Kidney Diseases. Cushing's syndrome, posted 1 June 2002. <http://endocrine.niddk.nih.gov/pubs/cushings/cushings.htm> (21 May 2006).

National Institute of Environmental Health Sciences. NIEHS PR #05-01. 31 January 2005a. <http://www.niehs.nih.gov/oc/news/canceragents.htm> (29 March 2006).

National Institute of Environmental Health Sciences. The report on carcinogens, eleventh edition. 31 January 2005b. <http://ntp.niehs.nih.gov/ntp/roc/toc11.html> (29 March 2006).

National Institute of Neurological Disorders and Stroke. Arteriovenous malformations and other vascular lesions of the central nervous system fact sheet, updated 23 January 2006. <http://www.ninds.nih.gov/disorders/avms/detail_avms.htm> (10 July 2006).

National Research Council Canada. Technetium, posted March 25, 2003. <http://www.nrc-cnrc.gc.ca/education/elements/el/tc_e.html> (April 21, 2006).

Navarro Silvera, S.A., Miller, A.B. and Rohan, T.E. Risk factors for thyroid cancer: a prospective cohort study. Int. J. Cancer. 116 (2005): 433-438.

Neugut, A.I. et al. The epidemiology of cancer of the small bowel. Cancer Epidemiol. Biomarkers Prev. 3 (1998): 243-251.

NewsTarget.com. State-sponsored medical terrorism: Texas authorities arrest parents, kidnap their teenage daughter, and force her through chemotherapy against her will. 3 January 2006. <http://www.newstarget.com/z016387.html> (28 April 2006).

The New York Times, Homicide charges are recommended in misread pap test, 11 April 1995. <http://query.nytimes.com/gst/fullpage.html?sec=health&res=990CE 1D81338F932A25757C0A963958260> (26 June 2006).

Ng, A.K. et al. Second malignancy after Hodgkin's disease treated with radiation therapy with or without chemotherapy: long-term risks and risk factors, Blood 100 (2002): 1989-1996.

Ng, A.K. et al. Factors influencing treatment recommendations in early-stage Hodgkin's disease: a survey of physicians. Ann. Oncol. 15 (2004): 261-269.

Nicholson, A.A. et al. Treatment of malignant superior vena cava obstruction: metal stents or radiation therapy. J. Vasc. Interv. Radiol. 8 (1997): 781-788.

Nobler, M.P., Leddy, M.E. and Huh, S.H. The impact of palliative irradiation on the management of patients with acquired immune deficiency syndrome. J. Clin. Oncol. 5 (1987): 107-112.

Non-small Cell Lung Cancer Collaborative Group. Chemotherapy in non-small cell lung cancer: a meta-analysis using updated data on individual patients from 52 randomised clinical trials. Br. Med. J. 311 (1995): 899-909.

Noordijk, E.M. et al. Radiotherapy as an alternative to surgery in elderly patients with resectable lung cancer. Radiother. Oncol. 13 (1988): 83-89.

Nordlinger, B. and Rougier, P. Nonsurgical methods for liver metastases including cryotherapy, radiofrequency ablation, and infusional treatment: what's new in 2001? Curr. Opin. Oncol. 14 (2002): 420-423.

Nuchtern, J.G. Perinatal neuroblastoma. Semin. Pediatr. Surg. 15 (2006): 10-16.

Nutting, C. et al. Radiotherapy in the treatment of benign meningioma of the skull base. J. Neurosurg. 90 (1999): 823-827.

Ocular Oncology Service. Treatment, 2005. <http://www.retinoblastomainfo.com/pages/treatment.htm> (6 July 2006.)

Ogawa, K. et al. Treatment and prognosis of thymic carcinoma: a retrospective analysis of 40 cases. Cancer 94 (2002): 3115-3119.

Oh, J.L. et al. Induction chemotherapy followed by concomitant chemoradiotherapy in the treatment of locoregionally advanced nasopharyngeal cancer. Ann. Oncol. 14 (2003): 564-569.

Olgac, S. et al. Urothelial carcinoma of the renal pelvis: a clinicopathologic study of 130 cases. Am. J. Surg. Pathol. 28 (2004): 1545:1552.

Olsen, O. and Gotzsche, P.C. Cochrane Review on screening for breast cancer with mammography. Lancet 358 (2001): 1340-1342.

Ormsby, M.V. et al. Wound complications of adjuvant radiation therapy in patients with soft-tissue sarcomas. Ann. Surg. 210 (1989): 93-99.

Ott, K. et al. Neoadjuvant chemotherapy with cisplatin, 5-FU, and leucovorin (PLF) in locally advanced gastric cancer: a prospective phase II study. Gastric Cancer 6 (2003): 159-167.

Ozols, R.F. et al. Phase III trial of carboplatin and paclitaxel compared with cisplatin and paclitaxel in patients with optimally resected stage III ovarian cancer: a gynecologic oncology group study. J. Clin. Oncol. 21 (2003): 3194-3200.

Paliwal, B.R., Brezovich, I.A. and Hendee, W.R. IMRT may be used to excess because of its higher reimbursement from Medicare. Med. Phys. 31 (2004): 1-3.

Parekh, S. Ratech and H. Sparano, J.A. Human immunodeficiency virus-associated lymphoma. Clin. Adv. Hematol. Oncol. 1 (2003): 295-301.

Pastorino, U. Early detection of lung cancer. Respiration 73 (2006): 5-13.

Paszat, L.F. et al. 1999. Mortality from myocardial infarction after adjuvant radiotherapy for breast cancer in the surveillance, epidemiology, and end-results cancer registries. J Clin. Oncol. 16 (1999): 2625-2631. See erratum in J. Clin. Oncol. 17 (1999) :740.

Patel, P.H., Chaganti, R.S. and Motzer, R.J. Targeted therapy for metastatic renal cell carcinoma. Br. J. Cancer 94 (2006): 614-619.

Patz, E.F., Jr. Swensen, S.J. and Herndon II, J.E. Estimate of lung cancer mortality from low-dose spiral computed tomography screening trials: implications for current mass screening recommendations. J. Clin. Oncol. 22 (2004): 2202-2206.

Paulussen, M. Frohlich and B. Jurgens, H. Ewing tumour: incidence, prognosis and treatment options. Paediatr. Drugs 12 (2001): 899-913.

Pavlidis, N. et al. Diagnostic and therapeutic management of cancer of an unknown primary. Eur. J. Cancer 39 (2003): 1990-2005.

Payne, D.M. Statement of congressman Donald Payne prostate cancer initiative, 19 March 2002.

<http://www.house.gov/list/press/nj10_payne/20020319prostate.htm
l> (24 June 2006).
Pectasides, D., Pectasides, M. and Economopoulos, T. Merkel cell
cancer of the skin. Ann. Oncol. (2006): epub
Pederson, L.C. and Lee, J.E. 2003. Pheochromocytoma. Curr. Treat.
Options Oncol. 4 (2003): 329-337.
Perez, C.A. et al. Definitive irradiation in carcinoma of the vagina: long-
term evaluation of results. Int. J. Radiat. Oncol. Biol. Phys. 15
(1988): 1283-1290.
Perez, C.A. et al. Irradiation in carcinoma of the vulva: factors affecting
outcome. Int. J. Radiat. Oncol. Biol. Phys. 42 (1998): 335-344.
Perez, C.A. et al. Factors affecting long-term outcome of irradiation in
carcinoma of the vagina. Int. J. Radiat. Oncol. Biol. Phys. 44 (1999):
37-45.
Pernot, M. et al. Iridium-192 brachytherapy in the management of 147
T2No oral tongue carcinomas treated with irradiation alone:
comparison of two treatment techniques. Radiother. Oncol. 23
(1992): 223-228.
Peschel, R. and Peschel, E. Guilt-in the company of Puccini's doctor.
Psychol. Rep. 66 (1990): 267-271,
Peschel, R.E. and Colberg, J.W. Surgery, brachytherapy, and external-
beam radiotherapy for early prostate cancer. Lancet Oncol. 4
(2003): 233-241.
Pierce, D.A. and Preston, D.L. Cancer risks at low doses among A-
bomb survivors. Radiat. Res. 15, Spring-Summer 2001.
Pignon, J.P. et al. A meta-analysis of thoracic radiotherapy for small-
cell lung cancer. N. Engl. J. Med. 327 (1992): 1618-1624.
Pisano, E.D. et al. Diagnostic performance of digital versus film
mammography for breast-cancer screening. N. Engl. J. Med. 353
(2005): 1773-1783.
Po Wing Yuen, A. et al. Prognostic factors of clinically stage I and II
oral tongue carcinoma - a comparative study of stage, thickness,
shape, growth pattern, invasive front malignancy grading, Martinez-
Gimeno score, and pathologic features. Head Neck 24 (2002): 513-
520.
Pogoda, J.M. and Preston-Martin, S. Solar radiation, lip protection, and
lip cancer risk in Los Angeles County women (California, United
States). Cancer Causes Control. 7 (1996): 458-463.
Pollack, A. et al. Prostate cancer radiation dose response: results of
the M. D. Anderson phase III randomized trial. Int. J. Radiat. Oncol.
Biol. Phys. 53 (2002): 1097-1105.
Pollack, A. et al. Radiation therapy dose escalation for prostate cancer:
a rationale for IMRT. World J. Urol. 21 (2003): 200-208.

Pollock, B.E., Gorman, D.A. and Brown, P.D. Radiosurgery for arteriovenous malformations of the basal ganglia, thalamus, and brainstem. J. Neurosurg. 100 (2004): 210-214.

Pollack, B.E. and Ecker, R.D. A prospective cost-effectiveness study of trigeminal neuralgia surgery. Clin. J. Pain 21 (2005): 317-322.

PORT Meta-analysis Trialists Group. Postoperative radiotherapy in non-small-Cell lung cancer: systematic review and meta-analysis of individual patient data from nine randomised controlled trials. Lancet 352 (1998): 257-263.

Poston, G.J. Naive interpretation of the data. A rapid response to Gottlieb, S., Resectable pancreatic cancer needs surgery, then chemotherapy. Br. Med. J. 328 (2004) :661.

Pow-Sang, M.R., et al. Cancer of the penis. Cancer Control 9 (2002): 305-314.

Proietti, F.A. et al. Global epidemiology of HTLV-I infection and associated diseases. Oncogene 24 (2005): 6058-6068.

Prosnitz, R.G. and Marks, L.B. Radiation-induced heart disease: vigilance is still required. J. Clin. Oncol. 23 (2005): 7391-7394.

Pui, C.H. et al. Rationale and design of total therapy study XV for newly diagnosed childhood acute lymphoblastic leukemia. Ann. Hematol. 83 (2004): S124-S126.

Puthawala, A.A. et al. Long-term results of treatment for prostate carcinoma by staging pelvic lymph node dissection and definitive irradiation using low-dose rate temporary iridium-192 interstitial implant and external beam radiotherapy. Cancer 92 (2001): 2084-2094.

Quivey, J.M. et al. High intensity 125-Iodine (125I) plaque treatment of uveal melanoma. Int. J. Radiat. Oncol. Biol. Phys. 26 (1993): 613-618.

Raffetto, N. et al. Radiotherapy alone and chemoirradiation in recurrent squamous cell carcinoma of the vulva. Anticancer Res. 23 (2003): 3105-3108.

Ragel, B. and Jensen, R.L. New approaches for the treatment of refractory meningiomas. Cancer Control. 14 (2003): 148-158.

Randall, M.E., Spirtos, N.M. and Dvoretsky, P. Whole abdominal radiotherapy versus combination chemotherapy with doxorubicin and cisplatin in advanced endometrial carcinoma (phase III): Gynecologic Oncology Group Study No. 122. J. Natl. Cancer Inst. Monogr. 19 (1995): 13-15.

Randi, G., Franceschi, S. and La Vecchia, C. Gallbladder cancer worldwide: geographical distribution and risk factors. Int. J. Cancer 118 (2006): 1591-1602.

Rao, A.V., Akabani, G. and Rizzieri, D.A. Radioimmunotherapy for non-Hodgkin's lymphoma. Clin. Med. Res. 3 (2005): 157-165.

Reddy, S.P. et al. Tumors of the uterine corpus, posted 1997. <http://www.cancernetwork.com/textbook/morev25.htm> (2 June 2006).

Reeder, C.E. and Gordon, D. Managing oncology costs. Am. J. Manag. Care 12 (2006): S3-S16.

Regis, J. et al. Gamma knife surgery in mesial temporal lobe epilepsy; a prospective multicenter study. Epilepsia 45 (2004): 504-515.

Resbeut, M.R. et al. Combined brachytherapy and surgery for early carcinoma of the uterine cervix: analysis of extent of surgery on outcome. Int. J. Radiat. Oncol. Biol. Phys. 50 (2001): 873-881.

Ries, L.A.G. et al., ed. Cancer incidence and survival among children and adolescents: United States SEER Program 1975-1995, National Cancer Institute, SEER program. NIH pub. no. 99-4649. Young, J.L., Jr. et al. Chapter V retinoblastoma, 1999.

Ries, L.A.G. et al., ed. SEER cancer statistics review, 1975-2003, based on November 2005 SEER data submission, posted to the SEER web site, 2006. <http://seer.cancer.gov/csr/1975_2003/> (8 June 2006).

Robertson, J.M. et al. Long-term results of hepatic artery fluorodeoxyuridine and conformal radiation therapy for primary hepatobiliary cancers. Int. J. Radiat. Oncol. Biol. Phys. 37 (1997): 325-330.

Rodriquez-Galindo, C. et al. Treatment of metastatic retinoblastoma. Ophthalmology 110 (2003): 1237-1240.

Rodriguez-Galindo, C. Pharmacological management of Ewing sarcoma family of tumours. Expert Opin. Pharmacother. 5 (2004): 1257-1270.

Roos, D.E. et al. Randomized trial of 8 G in 1 versus 20 Gy in 5 fractions of radiotherapy for neuropathic pain due to bone metastases (Trans-Tasman Radiation Oncology Group, TROG 96.05). Radiother. Oncol. 75 (2005): 54-63.

Rosenberg, M., Zerris, V. and Borden, J. Gamma knife radiosurgery for treatment of trigeminal neuralgia. J. Mass. Dent. Soc. 50 (2001): 40-43, 49.

Rosenblatt, K.A. et al. Marijuana use and risk of oral squamous cell carcinoma. Cancer Res. 64 (2004): 4049-4054.

Rosti, G. et al. Chemotherapy advances in small cell lung cancer. Ann Oncol. Suppl 5 (2006): 99-102.

Rouberol, F. et al. Survival, an atomic, and functional long-term results in choroidal and ciliary body melanoma after ruthenium brachytherapy (15 years' experience with beta rays). Am. J. Ophthalmol. 137 (2004): 893-900.

Rubie, H. et al. Localized and unresectable neuroblastoma in infants: excellent outcome with primary chemotherapy. Neuroblastoma Study Group, Societe Francaise d'Oncologie Pediatrique. Med. Pediatr. Oncol. 36 (2001): 247-250.

Rutkowski, T. et al. Efficacy and toxicity of MDR versus HDR brachytherapy for primary vaginal cancer. Neoplasma 49 (2002): 197-200.

Rutqvist, L.E. and Johansson, H. Mortality by laterality of the primary tumour among 55,000 breast cancer patients from the Swedish Cancer Registry. Br. J. Cancer 61 (1990): 866-888.

Rutqvist, L.E., Rose, C. and Cavallin-Stahl, E. A systematic overview of radiation therapy effects in breast cancer. Acta Oncol. 42 (2003): 532-545.

Sachdeva, K. et al. Renal cell carcinoma, updated December 29, 2005. <http://www.emedicine.com/med/topic2002.htm> (June 5, 2006).

Sadetzki, S. et al. Long-term follow-up for brain tumor development after childhood exposure to ionizing radiation for tinea capitis. Radiat Res. 163 (2005): 424-432.

Safioleas, M. et al. Diagnosis and treatment aspects of medullary thyroid carcinoma. Chirurgia (Bucur.) 101 (2006): 121-126.

Saif, M. W., Targeted agents for adjuvant therapy of colon cancer. Clin Colorectal Cancer 6 (2006): 46-51.

Sasaoka, M. et al. Patterns of failure in carcinoma of the uterine cervix treated with definitive radiotherapy alone. Am. J. Clin. Oncol. 24 (2003): 586-590.

Sause, W.T. et al. Radiation Therapy Oncology Group (RTOG) 88-08 and Eastern Cooperative Oncology Group (ECOG) 4588: preliminary results of a phase III trial in regionally advanced, unresectable non-small-cell lung cancer. J. Natl. Cancer Inst. 87 (1995): 198-205.

Sawyer, T.E. et al. Effectiveness of postoperative irradiation in stage IIIA non-small cell lung cancer according to regression tree analyses of recurrence risks. Ann. Thorc. Surg. 64 (1997): 1402-1407.

Schaake-Koning C. et al. Effects of concomitant cisplatin and radiotherapy on inoperable non-small-cell lung cancer. N. Engl. J. Med. 326 (1992): 524-530.

Schnirer, I.I., Yao, J.C. and Ajani, J.A. Carcinoid—a comprehensive review. Acta Oncol. 42 (2003): 672-692.

Scholz, M. and Holtl, W. Stage I testicular cancer. Curr. Opin. Urol. 13 (2003): 473-476.

Scutt, D., Lancaster, G.A. and Manning, J.T. Breast asymmetry and predisposition to breast cancer. Breast Cancer Res. 8 (2006): R14-R25.

Selch, M.T. et al. Stereotactic radiotherapy for treatment of cavernous sinus mengiomas. Int. J. Radiat. Oncol. Biol. Phys. 59 (2004): 101-111.

Semelka, R.C. Imaging X-rays cause cancer: a call to action for caregivers and patients, posted 13 February 2006, <http://www.medscape.com/viewprogram/5063_index> (29 May 2006).

Sengupta, S. and Zincke, H. Lessons learned in the surgical management of renal cell carcinoma. Urology 66 Suppl. 5 (2005): 36-42.

Serraino, D. et al. Infection with Epstein-Barr virus and cancer: an epidemiological review. J. Biol. Regul. Homeost. Agents 19 (2005): 63-70.

Sessions, D.G. et al. Analysis of treatment results for oral tongue cancer. Laryngoscope 112 (2002): 616-625.

Sessions, D.G. et al. Analysis of treatment results for base of tongue cancer. Laryngoscope 113 (2003): 1252-1261.

Sessions, D.G., Lenox, J. and Spector, G.J. Supraglottic laryngeal cancer: analysis of treatment results. Laryngoscope. 115 (2005): 1402-1410.

Shaha, A.R. Implications of prognostic factors and risk groups in the management of differentiated thyroid cancer. Laryngoscope 14 (2004): 393-402.

Sharma, P.K. and Johns, M.M. Thyroid cancer, updated 29 November 2004. <http://www.emedicine.com/ent/topic646.htm> (7 June 2006).

Shaw, et al. Radiation therapy in the management of low-grade supratentorial astrocytomas. J. Neurosurgery 70 (1989): 853-861.

Sherman, S.I. and Gopal, J. Thyroglobulin positive, RAI negative thyroid cancers: the role of conservative management. J. Clin. Endocrinol. Metab. 83 (1998): 4199-4200.

Shields, C.L. et al. Plaque radiotherapy for uveal melanoma: long-term visual outcome in 1106 consecutive patients. Arch. Ophthalmol. 118 (2000): 1219-1228.

Shields, C.L. et al. Plaque radiotherapy for retinoblastoma: long-term tumor control and treatment complications in 208 tumors. Opthalmology 108 (2001): 2116-2121.

Shikama, N. et al. Risk factors for local-regional recurrence following preoperative radiation therapy and surgery for head and neck cancer (stage II-IVB). Radiology 228 (2003): 789-794.

Shintani, T. et al. High incidence of meningioma among Hiroshima atomic bomb survivors. J. Radiat. Res. (Tokyo) 40 (1999): 49-57.

Shipley, J. et al. Phase III trial of neoadjuvant chemotherapy in patients with invasive bladder cancer treated with selective bladder preservation by combined radiation therapy and chemotherapy: initial results of Radiation Therapy Oncology Group 89-03. Clin. Oncol. 16 (1998): 3576-3583.

Shore, R.E. Radiation-induced skin cancer in humans, Med. Pediatr. Oncol. 36 (2001): 549-554.

Shrimpton, P.C. and Edyvean, S. CT scanner dosimetry. Br. J., Radiol. 71 (1998): 1-3.

Sifri, R. Gangadharappa, S. and Acheson, L.S. Identifying and testing for hereditary susceptibility to common cancers. CA Cancer J. Clin. 54 (2004): 309-326.

Singh, I. and Khaitan, A. Current trends in the management of carcinoma penis—a review. Int. Urol. Nephrol. 35 (2003): 215-225.

Skarin, A. and Dorfman, D.M. Non-Hodgkin's lymphomas: current classification and management. Cancer J. Clinicians 47 (1997): 351-372.

Slatkin, N. Cancer-related pain and its pharmacologic management in the patient with bone metastasis. J. Support Oncol. 4 Suppl. 2 (2006): 15-21.

Smalley, S.M. Breast implants and breast cancer screening. J. Midwifery Womens Health 48 (2003): 329-337.

Smith, R.S. et al. Treatment of high-risk uterine cancer with whole abdominopelvic radiation therapy. Int. J. Radiat. Oncol. Biol. Phys. 48 (2000): 767-778.

Smith-Bindman, R., et al. Comparison of screening mammography in the United States and the United Kingdom. J. Am. Med. Assoc. 290 (2003): 2129-2137.

Smith-Bindman, R. et al. Does utilization of screening mammography explain racial and ethnic differences in breast cancer? Ann. Intern. Med. 144 (2006): 541-553.

Sonne, J.E. and Schaefer, S.D. Supraglottic cancer, updated 21 August 2003. <http://www.emedicine.com/ent/topic687.htm> (6 June 2006).

Sonneveld, P. and Segeren, C.M. Changing concepts in multiple myeloma: from conventional chemotherapy to high-dose treatment. Eur. J. Cancer 39 (2003): 9-18.

Sontag, S. Illness as a metaphor & aids as a metaphor. Picador, 2001.

Speight, P.M. and Barrett, A.W. Salivary gland tumours. Oral Diseases 8 (2002): 229-240.

Spierer, M.M. et al. Tolerance of tissue transfers to adjuvant radiation therapy in primary soft tissue sarcoma of the extremity. Int. J. Radiat. Oncol. Biol. Phys. 56 (2003): 1112-1116.

Spreafico, F. et al. Intensive, very short-term chemotherapy for advanced Burkitt's lymphoma in children. J. Clin. Oncol. 20 (2002): 2783-2788.

Stahl, O. et al. The impact of testicular carcinoma and its treatment on sperm DNA integrity. Cancer 100 (2004): 1137-1144.

Stanford University Medical Center, interview by Lori Aratani. Job's rare variety of pancreas cancer one of most curable. San Jose Mercury News. 2 August 2004.

Steensma, D.P. and Bennett, J.M. The myelodysplastic syndromes: diagnosis and treatment. Mayo Clin. Proc. 81 (2006): 104-130.

Stein, M.E. et al. Radiation therapy in epidemic (African) Kaposi's sarcoma. Int. J. Radiat. Oncol. Biol. Phys. 27 (1993): 1181-1184.

Steinberg, G.D. et al. Bladder cancer, updated 3 November 2005. <http://www.emedicine.com/med/topic2344.htm> (5 June 2006).

Stewart, B.W. and Kleihues, P., ed. World cancer report. Lyon, France: IARC Press, 2003.

Stone, N.M. and Holden, C.A. Postirradiation angiosarcoma. Clin. Exp. Dermatol. 22 (1997): 46-47.

Stone, R.M., O'Donnell, M.R. and Sekeres, M.A. Acute myeloid leukemia. Hematology 1 (2004): 98-117.

Straatsma, B.R. Golden Jubilee Lecture. Randomized clinical trials of choroidal melanoma treatment. Indian J. Ophthalmol. 51 (2003): 17-23.

Straughn, J.M. et al. Stage IC adenocarcinoma of the endometrium: survival comparisons of surgically staged patients with and without adjuvant radiation therapy. Gynecol Oncol. 89 (2003): 295-300.

Stryker, J.A. Radiotherapy for vaginal carcinoma: a 23-year review. Br. J. Radiol. 73 (2000): 1200-1205.

Sun, E.C. et al. Salivary gland cancer in the United States. Cancer Epidemiol. Biomarkers Prev. 8 (1999): 1095-1100.

Surma-aho, O. et al. Adverse long-term effects of brain radiotherapy in adult low-grade glioma patients. Neurol. 56 (2001): 1285-1290.

Syed, A.M. et al. Long-term results of low-dose rate interstitial-intracavitary brachytherapy in the treatment of carcinoma of the cervix. Int. J. Radiat. Oncol. Biol. Phys. 54 (2002): 67-78.

Syrjänen, S. HPV infections and tonsillar carcinoma. J. Clin. Pathol. 57 (2004): 449-455.

Tabar, L. et al. Beyond randomized controlled trials: organized mammographic screening substantially reduces breast carcinoma mortality. Cancer 91 (2001): 1724-1731.

Tabone, M.D. et al. Outcome of radiation-related osteosarcoma after treatment of childhood and adolescent cancer: a study of 23 Cases. J. Clin. Oncol. 17 (1999): 2789-2795.

Tacev, T., Ptackova, B. and Strnad, V. Californium-252 (252Cf) versus conventional gamma radiation in the brachytherapy of advanced cervical carcinoma long-term treatment results of a randomized study. Strahlenther. Onkol. 179 (2003): 377-384.

Takehara, K. et al. Recurrence of invasive cervical carcinoma more than five years after initial therapy. Obstet. Gynecol. 98 (2001): 680-684.

Tarvainen, L. et al. Is the incidence of oral and pharyngeal cancer increasing in Finland? An epidemiological study of 17,383 cases in 1953-1999. Oral Dis. 10 (2004): 167-172.

Tateda M. et al. Management of the patients with hypopharyngeal cancer: eight-year experience of Miyagi Cancer Center in Japan. Tohoku J Exp Med. 205 (2005): 65-77.

Taylor, D.H., Jr. Van Scoyoc, L. and Hawley, S.T. Health insurance and mammography; would a Medicare buy-in take us to universal screening? Health Services Res. 37 (2002): 1469-1486.

Tewari, K.S. et al. Primary invasive carcinoma of the vagina: treatment with interstitial brachytherapy. Cancer 91 (2001): 758-770.

Tewari, K.S. and DiSaia, P.J. Radiation therapy for gynecologic cancer. J. Obstet. Gynaecol. Res. 28 (2002): 123-140.

Theta Reports. World mammography markets, product code: R151-139. April 2003.

Thoroddsen, A. et al. Spontaneous regression of pleural metastases after nephrectomy for renal cell carcinoma. Scand. J. Urol. Nephrol. 36 (2002): 396-398.

Tombolini, V. et al. Brachytherapy for squamous cell carcinoma of the lip. The experience of the Institute of Radiology of the University of Rome "La Sapienza". Tumori 84 (1998): 478-482.

Tombolini, V. et al. Radiotherapy in classic Kaposi's sarcoma (CKS): experience of the Institute of Radiology of University "La Sapienza" of Rome. Anticancer Res. 19 (1999): 4539-4544.

Tondini, C. et al. Combined modality treatment with primary CHOP chemotherapy followed by locoregional irradiation in stage I or II histologically aggressive non-Hodgkin's lymphomas. J. Clin. Oncol. 11 (1993): 720-725.

Touboul, E. et al. Adenocarcinoma of the endometrium treated with combined irradiation and surgery: study of 437 patients. Int. J. Radiat. Oncol. Biol. Phys. 50 (2001): 81-97.

Travis, L.B. et al. Second cancers among long-term survivors of non-Hodgkin's lymphoma, J. Natl. Cancer Inst. 85 (1993): 1932-1937.

Tsai, C.S. et al. The prognostic factors for patients with early cervical cancer treated by radical hysterectomy and postoperative radiotherapy. Gynecol. Oncol. 75 (1999): 328-333.

Tschudi, D., Stoeckli, S. and Schmid, S. Quality of life after different treatment modalities for carcinoma of the oropharynx. Laryngpscope 113 (2003): 1949-1954.

Tsina, E.K. et al. Treatment of metastatic tumors of the choroid with proton beam. Ophthalmology 112 (2005): 337-343.

Tung, H.T. et al. 1999. Risk factors for breast cancer in Japan, with special attention to anthropometric measurements and reproductive history. Jpn. J. Clin. Oncol. 29 (1999): 137-146.

U.S. Central Intelligence Agency. CIA world fact book, updated 6 June 2006. <http://www.cia.gov/cia/publications/factbook/index.html> (8 June 2006).

U.S. Census Bureau. Census 2000 data for the United States, revised 30 July 2003. <http://factfinder.census.gov/servlet/QTTable?_bm=y&-geo_id=01000US&-qr_name=DEC_2000_SF1_U_DP1&-ds_name=DEC_2000_SF1_U> (17 June 2006).

U.S. Department of Health and Human Services. Cancer and Asian/Pacific Islanders, modified 31 October 2005. <http://www.omhrc.gov/templates/content.aspx?ID=3055> (6 July 2006).

U.S. Environmental Protection Agency. Guidelines for carcinogen risk assessment, published in 51 FR 33992. 24 September 1986 and interim 1999.

U.S. Environmental Protection Agency. Integrated risk information system for vinyl chloride (CASRN 75-01-4). 7 August 2000. <http://www.epa.gov/iris/subst/1001.htm> (23 June 2006).

U.S. Environmental Protection Agency. Integrated risk information system for benzene (CASRN 71-43-2). 17 April 2003. <http://www.epa.gov/iris/subst/0276.htm> (23 June 2006).

U.S. Environmental Protection Agency. A citizen's guide to radon: the guide to protecting yourself and your family from radon, revised September 2005. <http://www.epa.gov/radon/pubs/citguide.html> (30 June 2006).

U.S. News and World Report. Best cancer hospitals 2005.

U.S. News and World Report. Best cancer hospitals 2006. 112, 17 July 2006.

Vakaet, Luc A.M.-L. and Boterberg, T. Pain control by ionizing radiation of bone metastasis. Int. J. Dev. Biol. 48 (2004): 599-606.

Vallières, E. Adjuvant radiation therapy after complete resection of non–small-cell lung cancer. J.Clin. Oncol. 20 (2002): 1427-1429.

van Berkel, A.M. et al. A prospective randomized trial of Tannenbaum-type Teflon coated stents versus polyethylene stents for distal malignant biliary obstruction. Eur. J. Gastroenterol. Hepatol. 16 (2004): 213-217.

van Roijen, L. et al. Costs and effects of microsurgey versus radiosurgery in treating acoustic neuroma. Acta Neurochir. (Wien) 139 (1997): 942-948.

van Ruth, S. Baas, P. and Zoetmulder, F.A.N., Surgical treatment of malignant pleural mesothelioma. Chest 123 (2003): 551-561.

Varia, M.A. et al. Intraperitoneal radioactive phosphorus (32P) versus observation after negative second-look laparotomy for stage III ovarian carcinoma: a randomized trial of the gynecologic oncology group. J. Clin. Oncol. 21 (2003): 2849-2855.

Varian Medical Systems. Varian Medical Systems reports that the number of centers offering SmartBeam IMRT more than doubled in 2001. 18 January 2002. <http://www.pancreatica.org/full_articles/f2002_01_08.html> (18 April 2004).

Varian Medical Systems, interview by Zina Moukheiber. Varian: the stealth health company. Forbes.com. 12 January 2004a.

Varian Medical Systems, interview by Matt Palmquist. Beaming in on the cure. SF Weekly. 28 April 2004b. <http://www.sfweekly.com/issues/2004-04-28/feature.html> (1 June 2006).

Varian Medical Systems. Varian Medical Systems announces expansion and new manufacturing facility in China. 25 May 2006. <http://biz.yahoo.com/prnews/060525/sfth004.html?.v=50> (14 June 2006).

Vaughan Hudson, B. et al. Clinical stage 1 non-Hodgkin's lymphoma: long-term follow-up of patients treated by the British National Lymphoma Investigation with radiotherapy alone as initial therapy. Br. J. Cancer 69 (1994): 1088-1093.

Verellen, D. and Vanhavere, F. Risk assessment of radiation-induced malignancies based on whole-body equivalent dose estimates for IMRT treatment in the head and neck region. Radiother. Oncol. 53 (1999): 199-203.

Vergote, I.B. et al. Randomized trial comparing cisplatin with radioactive phosphorus or whole-abdomen irradiation as adjuvant treatment of ovarian cancer. Cancer 69 (1992): 741-749.

Veronesi, U. et al. Breast conservation is a safe method in patients with small cancer of the breast. Long-term results of three randomised trials on 1,973 patients. Eur. J. Cancer 31A (1995): 1574-1579.

Villena Garrido, V. et al. Pleural mesothelioma: experience with 62 cases in 9 years. Archiv. Bronconeumol. 40 (2004): 203-208.

Vogelzang, N.J. et al. Phase III study of pemetrexed in combination with cisplatin versus cisplatin alone in patients with malignant pleural mesothelioma. J. Clin. Oncol. 21 (2003): 2636-2644.

von Schweinitz, D., Hero, B. and Berthold, F. The impact of surgical radicality on outcome in childhood neuroblastoma. Eur. J. Pediatr. Surg. 12 (2002): 402-409.

Vordermark, D. et al. Intracavitary afterloading boost in anal canal carcinoma. Results, function and quality of life. Strahlenther Onkol. 177 (2001): 252-258.

Walter, M.A. et al. Radioiodine therapy in hyperthyroidism: inverse correlation of pretherapeutic iodine uptake level and post-therapeutic outcome. Eur. J. Clin. Invest. 34 (2004): 365-370.

Warde, P. and Payne, D. Does thoracic irradiation improve survival and local control in limited-stage small-cell carcinoma of the lung? A meta-Analysis. J. Clin. Oncol. 10 (1992): 890-895.

Wartofsky, L. Management of patients with scan negative, thyroglobulin positive differentiated thyroid carcinoma. J. Clin. Endocrinol. Metab. 83 (1998): 4195-4199.

Watts, P. Retinoblastoma: clinical features and current concepts in management. J. Indian Med. Assoc. 101 (2003): 464-466.

Webb, S. The physical basis of IMRT and inverse planning. Br. J. Radiol. 76 (2003): 678-689.

Weirich, A. et al. Survival in nephroblastoma treated according to the trial and study SIOP-9/GPOH with respect to relapse and morbidity. Ann. Oncol. 15 (2004): 808-820.

Weiss, N.S. Breast cancer mortality in relation to clinical breast examination and breast self-examination. Breast J. 9 (2003): S86-S89.

Wernecke, E., interview by CNN.com. Parents lose custody bid for cancer-stricken daughter. 16 June 2005. <http://www.cnn.com/2005/LAW/06/16/medical.battle.ap> (16 June 2005).

Whitaker, J. Chemotherapy quotes. 5 April 2003. <http://www.ghchealth.com/chemotherapy-quotes.html> (2 June 2006).

Whitehead, R.P. et al. A phase II trial of vinorelbine tartrate in patients with disseminated malignant melanoma and one prior systemic therapy: a Southwest Oncology Group Study. Cancer 100 (2004): 1699-1704.

Whittington, R. et al. Multimodality therapy of localized unresectable pancreatic adenocarcinoma. Cancer 54 (1984): 1991-1998.

Wiest, P.W. et al. CT scanning: a major source of radiation exposure. Semin. Ultrasound CT MR, 23 (2002): 402-410.

Windhal, T. and Andersson, S.O. Combined laser treatment for penile carcinoma: results after long-term followup. J. Urol. 169 (2003): 2118-2121.

Witzig, T.E. Yttrium-90-ibritumomab tiuxetan radioimmunotherapy: a new treatment approach for B-cell non-Hodgkin's lymphoma. Drugs Today (Barc). 40 (2004): 111-119.

Wolden, S.L. et al. Intensity-modulated radiation therapy (IMRT) for nasopharynx cancer: update of the Memorial Sloan-Kettering experience. 64 (2006): 57-62.

Wolmark, N. et al. Randomized trial of postoperative adjuvant chemotherapy with or without radiotherapy for carcinoma of the rectum: National Surgical Adjuvant Breast and Bowel Project Protocol R-02. J. Natl. Cancer Inst. 92 (2000): 388-396.

Wong, F.L. et al. Cancer incidence after retinoblastoma. Radiation dose and sarcoma risk. J. Am. Med. Assoc. 278 (1997): 1262-1267.

Wong, R.H. et al. Interaction of vinyl chloride monomer exposure and hepatitis B. viral infection on liver Cancer. J. Occup. Environ. Med. 45 (2003): 379-383.

Woodward, W.A. et al. Cardiovascular death and second non-breast cancer malignancy after postmastectomy radiation and doxorubicin-based chemotherapy. Int. Radiat. Oncol. Biol. Phys. 57 (2003): 327-335.

World Health Organization. Smoking statistics. 28 May 2002. <http://www.wpro.who.int/media_centre/fact_sheets/fs_20020528.ht m> (6 June 2006).

World Health Organization. Global cancer rates could increase by 50% to 15 million by 2020. 3 April 2003. <http://www.who.int/mediacentre/news/releases/2003/pr27/en/print. html> (1 June 2006).

World Health Organization. Projections of mortality and burden of disease to 2030, annex table A-8. 17 October 2005a. <http://www3.who.int/whosis/menu.cfm?path=evidence,burden,burd en_proj,burden_proj_results&language=english> (19 June 2006).

World Health Organization. 50 facts: global health situation and trends 1955-2025. 25 November 2005b. < http://www.who.int/whr/1998/media_centre/50facts/en/> (24 March 2006).

WorldNetDaily.com. Radioactive prostate sets off airport alert. 14 April 2004. <http://www.worldnetdaily.com/news/article.asp?ARTICLE_ID=3802 0> (21 April 2004).

Yalman, D. et al. Evaluation of morbidity after external radiotherapy and intracavitary brachytherapy in 771 patients with carcinoma of the uterine cervix or endometrium. Eur. J. Gynaecol. Oncol. 23 (2002): 58-62.

Yamada, T. et al. High-dose-rate interstitial brachytherapy of Bartholin's gland: a case report. Gynecol. Oncol. 77 (2000): 193-196.

Yamazaki, H. et al. Lymph node metastasis of early oral tongue cancer after interstitial radiotherapy. Int. J. Radiat. Oncol. Biol. Phys. 58 (2004): 139-146.

Ye, W. et al. Helicobacter pylori infection and gastric atrophy: risk of adenocarcinoma and squamous-cell carcinoma of the esophagus and adenocarcinoma of the gastric cardia. J. Natl. Cancer Inst. 96 (2004): 388-396.

Yoshizawa, H. Hepatocellular carcinoma associated with hepatitis C virus infection in Japan: projection to other countries in the foreseeable future. Oncology. 1 (2002): 8-17.

Young, R.C. et al. Adjuvant treatment for early ovarian cancer: a randomized phase III trial of intraperitoneal 32P or intravenous cyclophosamide and cisplatin--a gynecologic oncology group study. J. Clin. Oncol. 21 (2003): 4350-4355.

Zagars, G.K., Goswitz, M.S. and Pollack, A. Liposarcoma: outcome and prognostic factors following conservation surgery and radiation therapy. Int. J. Radiat. Oncol. Biol. Phys. 36 (2003): 311-319.

Zagars, G.K. et al. Mortality after cure of testicular seminoma. J. Clin. Oncol. 22 (2004): 640-647.

Zahm, S.H. and Devesa, S.S. Childhood cancer: overview of incidence trends and environmental carcinogens. Environ. Health Perspect. 103 (1995): 177-184.

Zanzonico, P. Rothenberg, L.N. and Strauss, H.W. Radiation exposure of computed tomography and direct intracoronary angiography: risk has its reward. J. Am. Coll. Cardiol. 47 (2006): 1846-1849.

Zar, N. et al. Long-term survival of patients with small intestinal carcinoid. World J. Surg. 28 (2004): 1163-1168.

Zelefsky, M.J. et al. High-dose intensity modulated radiation therapy for prostate cancer: early toxicity and biochemical outcome in 772 patients. Int. J. Radiat. Oncol. Biol. Phys. 53 (2002): 1111-1116.

Zidan, J. et al. Treatment of Kaposi's sarcoma with vinblastine in patients with disseminated dermal disease. Isr. Med. Assoc. J. 3 (2001): 251-253.

Zimmermann, F.B. et al. Sequential and/or concurrent hypofractionated radiotherapy and concurrent chemotherapy in neoadjuvant treatment of advanced adenocarcinoma of the pancreas. Outcome and patterns of failure, Hepatogastroenterology 51 (2004): 1842-1846.

Zouhair, A. et al. Radiation therapy alone or combined surgery and radiation therapy in squamous-cell carcinoma of the penis? Eur. J. Cancer 37 (2001): 198-203.

Zouhair, A. et al. Decreased local control following radiation therapy alone in early-stage glottic carcinoma with anterior commissure extension, Strahlenther. Onkol. 180 (2004): 84-90.

Index